E P I D E M

PDQ™ Series

Claude A. Villee Jr., Ph.D., Editor

Johnson
PDQ Pharmacology

Kamoun et al
PDQ Biochemistry

Norman, Streiner
PDQ Statistics

Streiner, Norman, Munroe Blum
PDQ Epidemiology

PDQ (Pretty Darned Quick)

EPIDEMIOLOGY

DAVID L. STREINER, Ph.D., C. Psych.

Professor of Clinical Epidemiology and Biostatistics
and of Psychiatry

GEOFFREY R. NORMAN, Ph.D.

Professor of Clinical Epidemiology and Biostatistics

HEATHER MUNROE BLUM, Ph.D.

Assistant Professor of Psychiatry

all of
McMaster University Faculty of Health Sciences
Hamilton, Ontario

1989   B.C. Decker Inc • Toronto • Philadelphia

Publisher

B.C. Decker Inc
3228 South Service Road
Burlington, Ontario   L7N 3H8

B.C. Decker Inc
320 Walnut Street
Suite 400
Philadelphia, Pennsylvania   19106

Sales and Distribution

United States and Possessions	**The C.V. Mosby Company** 11830 Westline Industrial Drive Saint Louis, Missouri 63146
Canada	**The C.V. Mosby Company, Ltd.** 5240 Finch Avenue East, Unit No. 1 Scarborough, Ontario M1S 4P2
United Kingdom, Europe and the Middle East	**Blackwell Scientific Publications, Ltd.** Osney Mead, Oxford OX2 OEL, England
Australia	**Harcourt Brace Jovanovich** 30–52 Smidmore Street Marrickville, N.S.W. 2204 Australia
Japan	**Igaku-Shoin Ltd.** Tokyo International P.O. Box 5063 1–28–36 Hongo, Bunkyo-ku, Tokyo 113, Japan
Asia	**Info-Med Ltd.** 802–3 Ruttonjee House 11 Duddell Street Central Hong Kong
South Africa	**Libriger Book Distributors** Warehouse Number 8 "Die Ou Looiery" Tannery Road Hamilton, Bloemfontein 9300
South America (non-stock list representative only)	**Inter-Book Marketing Services** Rua das Palmeriras, 32 Apto. 701 222–70 Rio de Janeiro RJ, Brazil

PDQ Epidemiology   ISBN 1-55664-073-0

Library of Congress catalog card number: 88-51295

10   9   8   7   6   5   4

To
Betty, Steven, Lisa, Scott, Heather, & Shoshana
and
Pam, Leigh, & Adam
and
Lenny & Sydney

PREFACE

Welcome to the wonderful world of epidemiology. Just when you figured that you had mastered the mysteries of pulmonary blood flow, cardiac rhythms, electrolyte balance, gut motility, and cerebral anatomy, along came this strange guy in a tweed jacket muttering formulas, statistics, and foreign-sounding words like "relative risk," "positive predictive value," and "Mantel-Haenzel chi-square." He didn't look like a scientist; no dirty lab coat, scientific calculator, or long hair. He didn't look like a real doctor either; no clean lab coat, stethoscope, or designer length hair. Yet he had the arrogance to claim that he is both a clinician and a scientist—he is a Clinical Epidemiologist. Amid the hushed silence in the room you can overhear desperate whispers of, "What in the world is a clinical whatever-it-is-ologist?"

More particularly, why, in a world already overpopulated by physiologists, pharmacologists, pathologists, gerontologists, nephrologists, cardiologists, neurologists, and a dozen other relatively legitimate art forms, do we need yet another -ologist?

The answer, it seems, is that somewhere in that complex, compartmentalized world that lays claim to the human body as an object of study, common sense got lost in the shuffle. The reality is that, despite a tremendous explosion in biomedical science, we still know embarrassingly little about the workings of ourselves. No one knows the cause of most diseases, or the cure for that matter. No one can lay claim to the crystal ball that will predict accurately who, among a group of cancer or post-myocardial infarction patients, will survive a year. As a result, there is a considerable gap between the exact findings of the laboratory and the uncertain world of clinical medicine. This leaves enormous room for the dissemination of well-intended but useless tests, therapies, or theories. Some examples may illustrate the point:

1. As we have been told by the media on countless occasions, dioxin is about the most lethal chemical known. A tiny dose causes mice to curl up and die; dioxins are teratogenic, mutagenic, and carcinogenic in the lab. Yet, despite all the tons of Agent Orange dumped over Vietnam and some large spills in places like Seveso, Italy, there is no evidence that they are a significant human carcinogen.

2. Conversely, cigarette smoking is easily the most lethal human carcinogen, measured in the number of lives lost. Yet it was long after good scientific evidence from human studies convinced everyone (except tobacco farmers and cigarette manufacturers) that it caused cancer that scientists were able to induce cancers in mice in the laboratory.

3. Clofibrate was a very popular lipid-reducing agent in the mid-1960s. There was abundant laboratory evidence that it would work as

claimed. Unfortunately, later randomized trials proved that the drug killed more people than it saved.

4. We like to think that the days of patent medicines and snake oil sales-men have passed. (However, one visit to your local drugstore to peruse the over-the-counter antiarthritis drugs, none of which con-tains anything more than aspirin and all of which cost 10 times as much, should dispel that myth.) Nevertheless, mainstream medicine is still susceptible to the legitimate and honest claims of success of new therapies based on experience with few patients. Many of these therapies are eventually proved to have no value. One case in point is gastric freezing. There were a number of case reports, involving a total of about 1,500 patients, that indicated that it would cure ulcers. It was only later that trials demonstrated that the proce-dure was useless.

5. Whatever happened to tonsillectomies? It seems as if five out of six adults over the age of 40 had their tonsils removed in childhood, but very few of our children have to endure this agony. Credit for the turnaround belongs to one of the neater epidemiologic studies. It was common wisdom in those days that roughly half of all kids needed their tonsils removed. These investigators started with about 400 kids who still had their tonsils, and shipped them around to a group of respected physicians. Sure enough, 45 percent of tonsils had to go. The researchers removed these "diseased" kids from the study and sent the remaining ones around again (to different physi-cians, of course). This time 46 percent of the tonsils were slated to go. Now, the kids who were left (who had been judged healthy by two sets of physicians by this time) were marched before a third group of doctors. Want to guess how many were said to need ton-sillectomies? You got it—44 percent.

These examples nicely illustrate the role of epidemiology these days—it comfortably fills the gaping chasm between the scientific wis-dom of the wet laboratory and the clinical wisdom of the ward. The good news is that it isn't all that hard. Despite the fancy terminology, epidemi-ology is, above all, the science of common sense. (Its bedmate, biostatis-tics, isn't quite so straightforward. To decipher the arcane logic of statisticians, we heartily recommend another book in the *PDQ* series—*PDQ Statistics*. We're biased, of course, since we wrote it.)

The intent of this book is to translate the terminology of epidemiol-ogy into street talk, so that, we hope, the common sense of the methods will emerge. It's laid out a bit like a dictionary. Topics are grouped in logical, rather than alphabetic, order, so it would behoove you to tackle one section at a time. Chapter 1 is an introduction that goes into more detail about what epidemiology can and cannot do. Chapter 2 talks about experimental designs. Chapter 3 examines the issues in measurement, and Chapter 4 is devoted to the criteria of causation.

At the end of the second, third, and fourth chapters, we've provided guides to help you determine if articles that you have come across have made some basic mistakes in design or reasoning. As in our previous book, *PDQ Statistics*, we've called these illustrations "Convoluted Reasoning or Anti-Intellectual Pomposity Detectors," which we've abbreviated as "C.R.A.P. Detectors." This was done solely for the laudable purpose of conserving space, and anyone who reads any other meaning into this name reveals a low sense of humor; such people should enjoy this book.

We can't guarantee that your graduate degree will be mailed after you finish this book. Nevertheless, we hope that you will find all the fancy words a bit less intimidating.

REFERENCES

Bakwin H. Pseudodoxia pediatrica. N Engl J Med 1945; 232:691–697.

Miao LL. Gastric freezing: an example of the evaluation of medical therapy by randomized clinical trials. In: Bunker JP, Barnes BA, Mosteller F, eds. Costs, risks, and benefits of surgery. New York: Oxford University Press, 1977:198.

Oliver MF, Heady JA, Morris JN, Cooper J. W.H.O. cooperative trial on primary prevention of ischaemic heart disease using clofibrate to lower serum cholesterol: mortality follow-up. Lancet 1980; 2:379–385.

Serum dioxin in Vietnam-era veterans—preliminary report. MMWR 1987; 36:470–475.

CONTENTS

INTRODUCTION TO EPIDEMIOLOGY

DEFINITIONS

Contrary to popular belief, epidemiology is *not* the study of skin diseases — the root word is epidemic, not epidermis. By the way, if you really want to impress your friends, the word *epidemic* comes from the Greek *epi*, meaning "among," and *demos*, meaning "the people." Some scholar defined epidemiology as "the study of the distribution and determinants of health-related states and events in populations and the application of this study to the control of health problems," which no doubt is about as clear and self-evident as a mortgage contract.

Fortunately, recent history is on our side. Before Legionnaires' disease came along, the only people who had ever heard of epidemiology were other epidemiologists. Now with AIDS (acquired immunodeficiency syndrome) on the rise, epidemiology is tops on the list of careers advocated by every high school guidance counselor.

We still haven't told you what it really is. That's a deliberate sidestep on our part: Epidemiology covers a whole range of activities from surveys of disease outbreaks to randomized trials of new drugs. Some would argue that the common basis of all epidemiology is methods rather than content, in contrast to most scientific disciplines. Two features of the methods of epidemiology differentiate it from most other branches of medical science: (1) in epidemiology the unit of observation is generally *groups of people* rather than individuals or other objects such as molecules, cells, or mice, and (2) epidemiology is concerned with *comparisons* of one group of people with another. Epidemiologists are always muttering about the control group. The real reason for this is that, in the primitive world inhabited by epidemiologists, we can't make any really good predictions about how people should respond under a given set of conditions; we need a control group of folks who are alike in every way *except* the variable of interest to provide some basis for comparison. After all, most theories of science make quantitative predictions about the relationship among a set of variables. Epidemiologic predictions may concern, for example, the action of a drug, and take the form "Hypothesis 1: It works," or "Hypothesis 2: It doesn't work."

Modern epidemiology incorporates both classical or analytic-descriptive epidemiology and clinical epidemiology, as we describe in this chapter. As Cassel has noted, epidemiology is an example of a discipline that has usefully expanded beyond its initial boundaries (kind of like the Sahara desert).

CLASSICAL EPIDEMIOLOGY

Over 100 years ago when the term epidemiology was first introduced in the *Oxford English Dictionary*, it referred to studying epidemics. The focus was on the study of factors that cause or are associated with disease. In one early and classic example from the mid-1800s, John Snow, a British physician, investigated the causes of the increased rates of cholera in certain areas of London. He observed that the disease was most prevalent in districts supplied with water by the Lambeth Company and the Southwark and Vauxhall Company, both of which obtained their water from a section of the Thames River that was extremely polluted with sewage. He also noted that the rate of new cases of cholera declined in those parts of the city supplied by Lambeth Company after it relocated to a less polluted section of the Thames. At the same time there was no change in the incidence of the disease in areas supplied by the Southwark and Vauxhall Company, which continued to draw its water from the heavily polluted section of the Thames. Snow was aware that a variety of factors other than water source (such as socioeconomic status and housing conditions, among others) could account for the differences in rates of disease between the two geographic areas. Snow's brilliance lay in his recognition of an opportunity to test his hypothesis that drinking water from the Southwark and Vauxhall Company increased the risk of cholera compared with the water supplied by the Lambeth Company. In his book, *On the Mode of Communication of Cholera*, Snow noted that

> Each company supplies both rich and poor, both large houses and small; there is no difference either in the condition or the occupation of the persons receiving the water of the different companies . . . . The (natural) experiment, too, was on the grandest scale. No fewer than three hundred thousand people of both sexes, of every age and occupation, and of every rank and station, from gentle folks down to the very poor, were divided into two groups without their choice, and, in most cases, without their knowledge; one group being supplied with water containing the sewage of London and amongst it, whatever might have come from the cholera patients, the other group having water quite free from such impurity. To turn this grand experiment to account, all that was required was to learn the supply of water to each individual house where a fatal attack of cholera might occur.

Walking from door to door (who ever said epidemiology is an armchair profession?), Snow documented the source of drinking water for every house where a death from cholera had taken place. In this way he determined that the polluted water, supplied by the Southwark and Vauxhall Company, was indeed responsible for the cholera epidemic.

This descriptive and analytic role of epidemiology continues to be important today in describing patterns of health and disease in communities, in contributing to our understanding of the natural history and clinical course of disease, and in identifying causal relationships. Classical epidemiology, sometimes referred to as "Big E" epidemiology, is associated with specific research approaches that are described in *Research Methodology.*

PERSON, PLACE, AND TIME

Classical epidemiology is concerned with three major variables that describe the features of the distribution of a disease or other health-related state: person, place, and time.

Person characteristics include such factors as gender (what we used to call "sex"), age, race, marital status, and socioeconomic status, among others. For example, some conditions may occur with greater frequency in one racial group than another, such as sickle cell anemia among blacks, thalassemia among Greeks and Italians, and Tay-Sachs disease among European Jews. Racial differences in the distribution of a disease can suggest a genetic root in the origins of the disorder.

The *place* or geographic distribution of a health-related outcome of interest can also be of importance in, for instance, understanding causal relationships or planning health services to meet the needs of a particular community. Geographic differences can suggest a role for factors such as climate or cultural practices, including diet, methods of food preparation, and food storage, in the promotion of a particular disease. For example, geographic comparisons from 39 countries demonstrate a strong correlation between breast cancer mortality rates and the intake of dietary fat (Fig. 1-1).

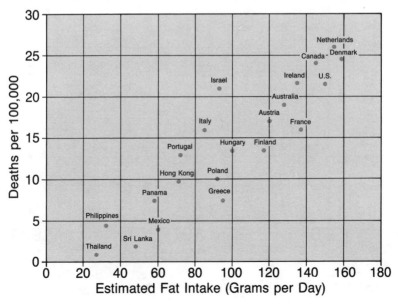

Figure 1-1   Geographic comparisons demonstrate a strong relationship between breast cancer mortality rates and the intake of dietary fat. (Data from Cohen LA. Diet and cancer. Sci Am 1987; 257:42-48.)

Variations in the *time* of occurrence of a particular disease can also indicate causal relationships among variables, although many different factors can account for the changes in disease distribution over time. For example, in many countries there has been a dramatic decline in the community incidence of dental caries over the past 20 years, which started with the gradual introduction of fluoride into community water systems, and of fluoride rinsing programs into the schools. Data from New Zealand show that a 12-year-old in 1971 would have had nine decayed, missing, or filled (DMF) teeth, whereas in 1983 the average 12-year-old had three DMF teeth (Fig. 1-2).

This strongly suggests a preventive role for fluoride, since no factors have been introduced simultaneously on such a massive scale that might otherwise explain the decline of tooth decay. This finding probably explains why more and more kids and Yuppies are wearing braces — dentists have to pay mortgages too!

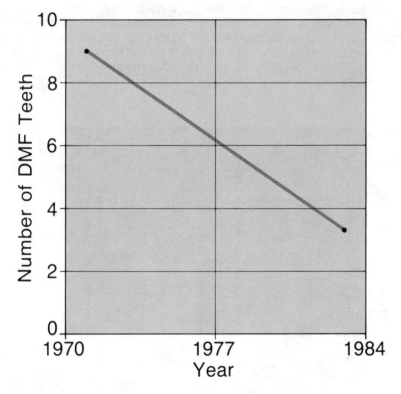

Figure 1-2   Time variable indicates causal relationship between decline in dental caries and the introduction of fluoride in New Zealand.

The variables of person, place, and time are important in understanding the nature of person-environment fit, a key construct in assessing the risk and protective factors that determine health status in groups of people.

CLINICAL EPIDEMIOLOGY

More recently, scientists such as Paul, Cassel, and Sackett and his colleagues, Feinstein, the Fletchers, and Wagner have formalized an additional branch of epidemiology termed **clinical epidemiology**. This approach applies the principles of epidemiology to the direct care of patients, sorting out research findings that are clinically useful from those that are primarily useful for tenure decisions. The hope is that this will result in more good and less harm to patients — a laudable goal.

CRITICAL APPRAISAL, DIAGNOSIS, AND MANAGEMENT

The behaviors of clinicians are based on their knowledge and beliefs about what actions are helpful in responding to a particular clinical problem; this knowledge may, in turn, be shaped by factors such as their prior experiences with similar problems, the advice of a trusted authority, and what they have read in scientific journals. These sources of information can lead to conclusions that may or may not be relevant, valid, and helpful in answering a particular clinical question. Clinical epidemiology offers clinicians specific criteria that can be applied to gauge the validity and usefulness of information they encounter when seeking to resolve a clinical problem. The buzzword for these criteria is **critical appraisal**.

TRENDS IN EPIDEMIOLOGY

As epidemiology has expanded to incorporate clinical decision making with classical or descriptive approaches, it has changed over time in regard to the nature of the diseases or health states with which it is concerned. The initial emphasis of epidemiology was on the study of infectious diseases of epidemic proportions, such as cholera and smallpox, at a time when communicable diseases plagued people everywhere and constituted the major health problem.

With improved hygiene and nutrition, advances in medical practice, and other factors, the major diseases have changed in most Western countries and are in a period of transition from infectious to chronic disease patterns in many developing nations. Epidemiology naturally followed this progression from its origins in the Age of Pestilence and Famine (infectious disease and starvation), through an Age of Receding Pandemics (decline in widespread epidemics), to an Age of Degenerative and Manmade Diseases (such as cancer, mental illness, occupational disorders, and cardiovascular disease).

About 1900 an eminent professor decreed that, given the natural history of physics, approximately 3 more years of research would solve all the remaining problems, but, in the process, he drastically underestimated the survival instincts of researchers. Epidemiologists have been equally adaptive, moving from infections to chronic diseases to drug trials (where the real money is!). However, in the last decade the wheel has come full circle with the onset of AIDS. As the disease spreads to pandemic proportions, it poses a new challenge to epidemiologists and other scientists (and guarantees many years of employment).

CURRENT APPLICATIONS OF EPIDEMIOLOGY

In case you're still confused about what this marvelous new (old) science is all about, this section provides some topical examples.

IDENTIFYING THE CAUSE OF A NEW SYNDROME

The late 1970s saw a number of cases of menstruating women who experienced a cluster of symptoms including fever, hypotension, and a rash that was followed by peeling of the skin. By 1980, 50 cases had been reported to the Centers for Disease Control in Atlanta and three women had died. Two questions required an urgent response: (1) Is this a new syndrome? and (2) What is causing it?

Through examination of the records, it was determined that these 50 cases were presenting a new clinical entity described by Langmuir as a "distinct clinical syndrome of marked severity and considerable clinical specificity." This syndrome was labeled "toxic shock syndrome."

The cause of the disease was established through a comparison of these women with a control group on a number of variables. There was no difference in their histories of sexually transmitted diseases, vaginal infections, frequency of intercourse, or intercourse during menstruation. On the other hand, 100 percent of the subjects used tampons, compared with 83 percent of the controls, and the women were significantly more likely to have used Rely brand tampons when compared with controls. That clinched it! In due course Rely brand tampons were withdrawn from the market.

This example demonstrates the strength of epidemiologic methods. Even given a relatively rare condition (toxic shock syndrome) associated with a very common practice (tampon use), it could nonetheless be established that tampon users had more than a tenfold greater risk of developing the condition compared with nontampon users.

ASSESSING THE RISKS ASSOCIATED WITH A HARMFUL EXPOSURE

Epidemiologic methods can be used to assess the risks to health that result from exposure to noxious agents. For example, with the worldwide use of nuclear reactors to generate power, the public, the nuclear power industry, and nuclear regulatory bodies are all extremely interested (obviously for different reasons) in determining the risks associated with exposure to the radioactive emissions resulting from a nuclear "accident" (a benign term for a malignant condition). These interests are not merely hypothetical or academic. In 1957 the first documented nuclear "accident," or substantial release of radioactivity from a nuclear power plant, occurred when a reactor caught fire at Sellafield on the Irish coast of Britain; in 1979 a nuclear accident occurred when a reactor was damaged at Three Mile Island; and in 1986 the most severe nuclear accident to date occurred at Chernobyl, in the USSR, when the graphite core of a reactor caught fire and caused the rupture or "meltdown" of fuel rods and the release of radioactive fission products into the atmosphere. Winds distributed the radioactive particles over large areas of Europe and the Northern Hemisphere.

It is of obvious importance to determine the immediate and long-term risks to the populations in the immediate vicinity of the accident and to those farther from the reactor (in other regions or countries). Fortunately, there is already a great deal of evidence available about the risks of cancer, childhood leukemia, birth defects, and so forth that result from exposure to high- and low-level radiation. By far the most extensive source of human evidence resulted from careful follow-up over the past 4 decades of the survivors of the Hiroshima and Nagasaki bombings. The basic strategy is to document, as carefully as possible, the radiation exposure of each individual and then compare the rate of onset of various diseases at different levels, from no exposure to a very high level. Other sources of evidence derive from the documented exposure of soldiers in the atom bomb tests of the 1950s, workers at the shipyards where nuclear submarines were serviced, populations exposed to the fallout clouds in Utah and Nevada, atomic workers, and even kids (now in their 40s) who put their feet in fluoroscopy machines at the local shoe store.

Based on this evidence, the scientists have predicted that there might be as many as 39,000 additional cancer deaths worldwide over the next 50 years. Since there are expected to be about 630 million deaths from cancer over the same period, the increase will not be detectable. Within the USSR, estimates range from 5,000 to 50,000 deaths against a background of 9.5 million cancer deaths; again, the difference would not be statistically significant. However, among the 24,000 people who lived within 15 km of the reactor site, the estimated excess number of cancers is 13, which raises the total to 624; this would be statistically detectable.

Epidemiologic studies have played a fundamental role in demonstrating the risk to health from such domestic exposures as smoking, nitrates in food, high dietary cholesterol, and occupational exposure to factors like asbestos, lead, and rubber. Conversely, epidemiologic methods have shown that there exists little evidence of harm from other exposures. For example, formaldehyde release from ureaformaldehyde foam insulation, "yellow rain" in Southeast Asia, video display terminals, and Love Canal have all, at one time or another, been featured prominently in news reports. Subsequent epidemiologic investigations, however, have revealed little in the way of measurable health problems from these highly publicized cases.

In turn, the identification of these risk factors may lead to the identification and effective treatment of those already exposed (e.g., screening and treatment for hypertension), and can suggest strategies for prevention (for example, guarantees of adequate income for single-parent families to prevent some childhood psychiatric disorders).

HOW TO DETERMINE IF A TREATMENT IS EFFECTIVE

You are a 33-year-old mother of two. Last week you noticed a small lump in one breast. With considerable apprehension you made an appointment with your family doctor. Today the doctor announced that your fear was justified; the lump is malignant.

Your physician is recommending total mastectomy (a surgical procedure that involves amputation of the breast, but not of the underlying muscle and lymph nodes), and assures you that if you have this procedure your condition is almost certainly curable. A friend of yours had a diagnosis of breast cancer over 1 year ago, and her physician removed just enough tissue to eliminate the tumor (segmental mastectomy) and gave her radiation therapy. You are frightened by the disease and want the treatment that will be most effective in preventing a recurrence of the cancer. On the other hand, you are devastated at the prospect of losing your breast. Clearly, if the treatment your friend had is as effective as total mastectomy, it would be your treatment of choice.

How do you decide what to do? Being human, you likely would seek out other friends who have gone through the procedures. In the absence of friends there is still *Family Circle* and *Consumer Reports* (the latter, actually, does a good job of reporting medical research). However, if you or your close friends had access to Medline and a medical library, there is the option of seeking out the original articles.

Clinical epidemiology figures prominently in the review. The methods of clinical epidemiology have contributed much to the assessment of the effectiveness of particular treatments. In the case of breast cancer the primary issue is whether there is any greater chance of survival with total versus segmental mastectomy. The question of effectiveness must be clearly defined, including both the specifics of the treatment and the particular cases to which it is applied. For example, segmental surgery may be just as effective in treating early stage breast cancer, whereas it may well be ineffective in treating later stage breast cancer after the malignant cells have spread beyond the immediate area.

Some additional concerns may relate to the side effects. If there is no difference in survival between two treatments, it becomes a tradeoff between the short-term discomfort from chemotherapy or hair loss from radiation against the disfigurement and disability from the loss of the breast. An approach that may help when examining side effects is to seek out information about the differences in psychological adjustment following total mastectomy versus segmental mastectomy and radiation therapy.

The best data on whether a treatment does more good than harm come from an experimental study design called the **randomized controlled trial (RCT)**. Here, patients with the disorder are randomly allocated to receive either the experimental treatment or conventional therapy (or a placebo), and then followed up so that the clinically relevant outcomes of the disease and treatment can be described and compared (see *Research Methodology* for more complete details of the RCT design). If you were the woman in our breast cancer example, and if, in an improbably objective frame of mind, you wanted to apply epidemiologic principles to determine the treatment of choice, you would want to know if any RCTs had been conducted comparing total mastectomy to more conservative surgery and radiation therapy.

As it turns out, there are several such trials. A recent one found that segmental mastectomy, with or without radiation, was superior to total mastectomy (Fig. 1-3). More women remained disease-free and more women were still alive 5 years after the procedure, whether or not the cancer had recurred. So, your literature search would give you the ammunition to say that segmental mastectomy not only is less disfiguring, but also likely leads to a better outcome.

HOW TO IDENTIFY HEALTH SERVICE UTILIZATION NEEDS AND TRENDS

Modern epidemiology plays an important role in the development of methods that can be used to describe health services and to test alternative ways to "deliver the goods." As an example, one often-debated health service question concerns the effect of health insurance coverage on the health services used by poor and near-poor populations. Conservatives claim that allowing people free access to health care services will open the

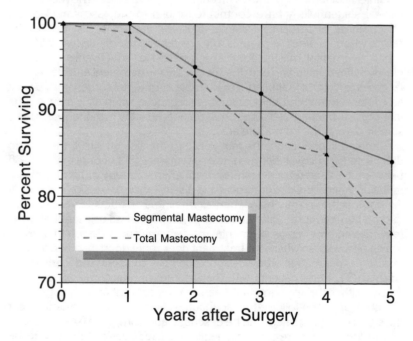

Figure 1-3 Data from a randomized controlled trial showing survival rates following segmental and total mastectomies.

floodgates and result in massive increases in health care costs. In so doing they ignore two kinds of data: (1) the several decades of experience in Canada and western Europe that provide ample demonstration that there is a practical ceiling on use of health services, and (2) the unpleasant experience of cooling one's heels in a doctor's waiting room, thumbing 10-year-old copies of *Reader's Digest*. The idea that people would prefer this to doing almost anything else is bizarre. By contrast, socialists live in their own version of utopia, where all are equal — in access, income, and reason. In socialist heaven no clear-thinking individual would dare to take undue advantage of free health care services, and utilization rates would not differ regardless of the method of payment.

Obviously, truth lies somewhere in between these extremes. Taube and Rupp conducted a study to assess the effect of Medicaid coverage on access to ambulatory mental health care for the poor and near-poor under 65 years of age. Analyzing data from the National Medical Care Utilization and Expenditure Survey, they found that the poor and near-poor with continuous Medicaid coverage used almost twice as much service as the poor and near-poor not enrolled in Medicaid (Fig. 1-4).

They concluded that the higher probability of use in those covered by Medicaid reflects the impact of the increased financial accessibility to needed mental health services. (This is a fine demonstration of the art of sciencemanship. Take an obvious and self-evident conclusion from the data, and clothe it in big obscure words so it sounds profound.)

This is only one example. Our personal favorite, which neatly skewers

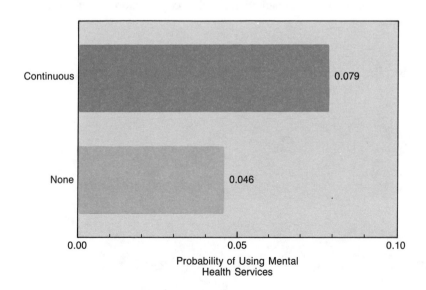

Figure 1-4 Data showing the effect of Medicaid coverage on access to ambulatory health care for the poor and near-poor populations under 65 years.

those who assume that every additional dollar spent on health care is a dollar well spent, is the repeated demonstration (in Scandinavia, Israel, and Canada) that when the doctors go on a protracted strike, the mortality rate drops.

Some other variations on this theme are *health economics*, which combines epidemiologic and economic methods to examine the cost-effectiveness of alternative models of delivery, and *policy analysis*, which seeks to link research findings to change in health policy.

SUMMARY

Epidemiology is a combination of knowledge and research methods concerned with the distribution and determinants of health and illness in populations, and with contributors to health and control of health problems. It comprises an analytic, descriptive component termed *classical epidemiology*, and a component concerned with critical appraisal of the research literature and diagnosis and management of illness, which is termed *clinical epidemiology*.

Modern epidemiology contributes to defining new clinical syndromes and their causes, as well as to completing the picture of the natural history and clinical course of a disease. It assists in the identification of the health risks associated with particular exposures and suggests strategies for disease prevention. It provides the criteria and methodology for determining if a treatment is effective and for describing and identifying health services needs and trends. Epidemiology has application to a range of health-related disciplines and has benefited from the contributions of a variety of professions.

REFERENCES

DEFINITIONS

Cassel JC. Community diagnosis. In: Omran AR, ed. Community medicine in developing countries. New York: Springer, 1974:345.

Last JM. A dictionary of epidemiology. Oxford: Oxford University Press, 1983.

MacMahon B, Pugh TF. Epidemiology: principles and methods. Boston: Little, Brown, 1970.

Oxford English Dictionary. London: Oxford University Press, 1971.

Cholera Example

Snow J. On the mode of communication of cholera. 2nd ed. London: Churchill, 1855. Reproduced in: Snow on cholera. New York: Commonwealth Fund, 1936.

Dietary Fat and Breast Cancer Example

Cohen LA. Diet and cancer. Sci Am 1987; 257:42-48.

Fluoride Example

Working Group of the Federation Dentaire Internationale and the World Health Organization. Changing patterns of oral health and implications for oral health manpower. I. Int Dent J 1985; 35:235-251.

Clinical Epidemiology

Fletcher RH, Fletcher SW, Wagner EH. Clinical epidemiology: the essentials. Baltimore: Williams & Wilkins, 1982.

Sackett DL, Haynes RB, Tugwell P. Clinical epidemiology: a basic science for clinical medicine. Toronto: Little, Brown, 1985.

TRENDS IN EPIDEMIOLOGY

Omran AR. Changing patterns of health and disease during the process of national development. In: Omran AR, ed. Community medicine in developing countries. New York: Springer, 1974:259.

CURRENT APPLICATIONS OF EPIDEMIOLOGY

Morris JN. Uses of epidemiology. New York: Churchill Livingstone, 1975.
Sackett DL, Haynes RB, Tugwell P. Clinical epidemiology: a basic science for clinical medicine. Toronto: Little, Brown, 1985.

Toxic Shock Syndrome

Helgerson SD, Foster LR. Toxic shock syndrome in Oregon: epidemiologic findings. Ann Intern Med 1982; 96(2):909-911.
Langmuir AD. Toxic shock syndrome — an epidemiologist's view. J Infect Dis 1982; 4:588-591.
Schlech WF, Shands KN, Reingold AL, et al. Risk factors for development of toxic shock syndrome: association with a tampon brand. JAMA 1982; 7:835-839.
Stallones RA. A review of the epidemiological studies of toxic shock syndrome. Ann Intern Med 1982; 96(2):917-920.

Nuclear "Accidents"

Ahearne J. Nuclear power after Chernobyl. Science 1987; 236:673-679.
Baverstock KF. A preliminary assessment of the consequences for inhabitants of the UK of the Chernobyl accident. Int J Radiat Biol 1986; 50:3-13.
Fernberg SE, Bromet EJ, Follman D, Lambert D, May SM. Longitudinal analysis of categorical epidemiological data: a study of Three Mile Island. Environ Health Perspect 1985; 63:241-248.

Ureaformaldehyde Foam Insulation

Norman GR, Newhouse MT. Health effects of ureaformaldehyde foam insulation: evidence of causation. Can Med Assoc J 1986; 134:733-737.

Strategies for Prevention

Munroe Blum H, Boyle MH, Offord DR. Single-parent families — child psychiatric disorder and school performance. J Am Acad Child Adolesc Psychiatry 1988; 27:214-219.
Offord DR. Prevention of behavioral and emotional disorders in children. J Child Psychol Psychiatry 1987; 28:9-19.

Treatment of Early Breast Cancer

Fisher BF, Bauer M, Margolese R, et al. Five-year results of a randomized clinical trial comparing total mastectomy and segmental mastectomy with or without radiation in the treatment of breast cancer. N Engl J Med 1985; 312:665-673.

Friedman NB. Mammary carcinoma and radiation therapy. Arch Surg 1987; 122:754-755.

Health Insurance Coverage

Taube CA, Rupp A. The effect of Medicaid on access to ambulatory mental health care for the poor and near-poor. Med Care 1986; 24:677-687.

TO READ FURTHER

Fletcher RH, Fletcher SW, Wagner EH. Clinical epidemiology: the essentials. Baltimore: Williams & Wilkins, 1982.

Henneckens CH, Buring JE. Epidemiology in medicine. Boston: Little, Brown, 1987.

MacMahon B, Pugh TF. Epidemiology: principles and methods. Boston: Little, Brown, 1970.

Omran AR. Changing patterns of health and disease during the process of national development. In: Omran AR, ed. Community medicine in developing countries. New York: Springer, 1974:259.

Sackett DL, Haynes RB, Tugwell P. Clinical epidemiology: a basic science for clinical medicine. Toronto: Little, Brown, 1985.

RESEARCH METHODOLOGY

In the early 1980s there was a flurry of articles in the popular press that reported the supposed hazards of video display terminals (VDTs) — those TV-like terminals connected to large computers or sitting on top of micro-computers. These purported adverse effects ranged from relatively mild ones like fatigue to more serious ones that affected pregnant women, such as stillbirths, miscarriages, and congenital fetal abnormalities. One news-paper reported that four of seven women who worked with VDTs gave birth to children with defects. This news story created a considerable stir and was cited in a Canadian task-force report on hazards in the workplace. Since anywhere between 1 million and 7 million people in North America use these terminals on a daily basis, they would represent a major health hazard were these reports true.

The task of the epidemiologist in this situation is twofold: (1) to determine if there is indeed an increased risk to the fetus caused by the mother working with VDTs; and (2) if so, to determine what the magnitude of that risk is. In this section we explore some of the possible research designs that could be used to answer these questions. We begin with the basic elements of research design; then discuss various factors, called **threats to validity**, that may lead us to draw erroneous conclusions from the data; and then show how the different design elements can be combined into various types of studies to minimize these threats to validity.

When discussing the different types of sampling strategies, biases, designs, and other elements our aim is not to be comprehensive; any such compendium is always incomplete, since the number of types is based solely on the imagination and inventiveness of the researcher. Rather, we mention some of the more common varieties of each of these factors to illustrate how they can be combined in various ways to address different issues.

DESIGN ELEMENTS

EXPERIMENTAL OR OBSERVATIONAL STUDIES

In **experimental** studies the intervention is under the control of the researcher. For example, the research team may determine (by random allocation) which subjects receive a novel treatment and which ones get traditional (or no) treatment, when an intervention is carried out in a community, or how much of a new drug each patient is given. The aim is to determine how changes in the **independent variable** (the one under the researcher's control) affect some outcome (the **dependent variable**). By controlling the timing or amount of the intervention, or which subjects get it and which ones do not, the chances are minimized that other factors outside of the researcher's control could have affected the results.

By contrast, the researcher does not control the intervention in **observational** studies, but rather observes the effects of an experiment in nature. It would be both unethical and impractical, for example, to expose some people to cigarette smoke or putative occupational carcinogens deliberately for 20 years to determine their effects. However, by choice or chance, some people have been exposed, so it is possible to draw some tentative conclusions based on observation of these subjects and, if possible, control subjects.

Most well-designed studies of a new treatment are experimental, in that the research team determines which subjects receive the new drug or intervention and which ones receive traditional treatment or a placebo. Almost all studies that involve exposure to harmful agents or that try to trace the natural history of a disorder are observational. However, these general rules naturally have exceptions. For example, if VDTs were being introduced gradually into the workplace, so that there were fewer terminals than eligible workers and there was no hard evidence of any adverse effects, women could be randomly assigned to work with them or remain using typewriters. However, this may be difficult to do because of practical considerations, and an observational type of study may be more realistic. (Needless to say, the researcher cannot control which women become pregnant. The last one who tried was hauled up on morality charges.)

NUMBER OF OBSERVATIONS

The simplest research design would involve looking at or measuring the outcome only once. In many cases, such as when the outcome is either present or absent or when the *timing* of the outcome is of minor interest, one observation may be all that is necessary. For example, if the question is whether working at a VDT results in a higher incidence of stillbirths, miscarriages, or congenital abnormalities, then we could record these outcomes 9 months after conception for this group of women and for an appropriate control group. The outcome is recorded only on a single occasion.

However, if we were interested in the *time course* of an outcome, one observation is not sufficient. To use a different example, Bagby and his colleagues looked at the effects of a new mental health act introduced toward the end of 1978 on the proportion of psychiatric patients who were involuntarily admitted to hospital (Fig. 2-1). The graph shows a dramatic decline in this type of admission following the new, more restrictive legislation. If the analysis had stopped at this point, it's likely that people would have come to the erroneous conclusion that the new act resulted in a reduction in the proportion of people being admitted to psychiatric wards on an involuntary basis. Multiple observations over time, however, show a different picture, that is, a gradual return to a level even higher than those of the 7 years preceding the new law. So, not only do multiple observations tell us something different than a single look does, they also reveal something about the "natural history" of the legislation; there was a gradual return to the previous mode of practice as psychiatrists learned to live with the new law.

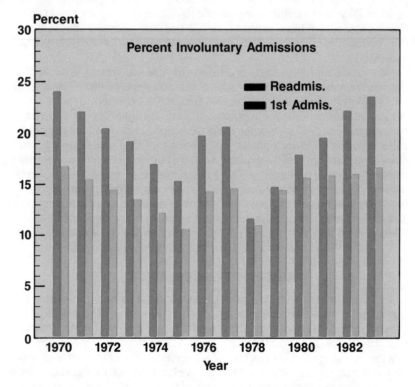

Figure 2-1 The proportion of psychiatric patients involuntarily admitted to hospital before and after the new mental health act of 1978.

DIRECTION OF DATA GATHERING

Data can be gathered in one of two ways: (1) looking *forward* and getting new data after the start of the study, or (2) looking *backward*, and using data that have already been collected. Specific names are used for each of these strategies. Studies that involve gathering data after the study has begun are called **prospective**; in **retrospective** studies the data have already been recorded for other reasons at some time in the past. The advantage of prospective data collection is that the nature of the data, the definitions of symptoms, the method by which the data are recorded, and other factors can be worked out ahead of time and are constant over the course of the trial. In retrospective studies definitions of symptoms or diseases may have been modified over time, units of measurement may have changed, and old methods for diagnosis may have been replaced, thereby resulting in more variability in the data. Perhaps the greatest advantage of prospective studies is that they allow us to determine the *directionality* of events (i.e., what occurred first and what happened later). As we'll see in *Assessing Causation*, this is necessary (but not sufficient) if we want to be able to say anything about causation. Information of this sort is far more difficult (some would say impossible) to obtain accurately in retrospective studies.

Doing the study retrospectively would involve identifying all women who were pregnant and worked with VDTs at least 9 months ago, and then either interviewing them or reviewing their hospital charts to determine the outcome of the pregnancy. This is advantageous because the study could be done relatively quickly, but it suffers from a few risks: the type of terminals may have changed, it may be difficult to establish how much time the women spent in front of the VDTs, and hospital documentation of all possible birth defects may be difficult to acquire (e.g., miscarriages may not have been recorded in hospital records.) A prospective study would enter women into the trial only if they became pregnant after the start date. Although the researcher could now record all the relevant information with greater accuracy, the study might have to continue for a few years until enough women became pregnant to allow analysis of the results.

The term "prospective" should *not* be used to describe trials in which historical data are gathered after a diagnosis or exposure that occurred some time in the past. For example, if we gather hospital utilization data from 1945 to the present on people who witnessed the A-bomb tests in Nevada, the data would still be retrospective, although the hospitalizations occurred after the exposure. Even though the subjects were followed forward in time, the data involve events that happened before *now*, and so the study would be called retrospective (Fig. 2-2).

A few authors have tried to clarify this confusion in nomenclature by introducing terms such as "retrolective," "prolective," or "retrospective-prospective." Laudable as this goal is, we feel that these neologisms have only further obfuscated the sufficiently murky picture.

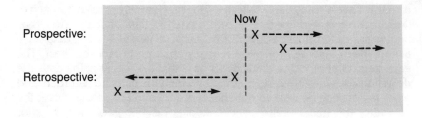

X   = When subject is enrolled in study

➤ = Direction of data gathering

Figure 2-2 Prospective versus retrospective studies.

COMPARISON GROUPS

Keeping with our study of women who worked with video display terminals, we could easily derive prevalence figures for each of the outcomes of interest (stillbirths, miscarriages, and congenital abnormalities), but the meaning of these numbers would be unclear. The major reason is that women who do *not* work in front of VDTs also experience these adverse effects.

So, now the question has become somewhat more complicated: Do women who work with VDTs have these outcomes *at a higher rate* than women who do not work in front of terminals? This means that we now need a group against which we can compare our prevalence results to determine if they are higher or not.

There are two major types of comparison or control groups: **historical** and **concurrent**. In the former case we would compare our results with data that already exist from previous studies (e.g., a large survey of the prevalence of miscarriages, stillbirths, and congenital abnormalities in the general population). If such data do not exist or if they are suspect for one reason or another, the researchers must gather information from a control group concurrently;   in essence, the researchers have at least two groups in the study.

When good historical control groups exist, they can save a considerable amount of time, effort, and expense. Unfortunately most historical control groups are compromised for some reason. The primary reason is that factors in the environment, such as clinical policies, may have changed since the data were originally gathered. For example, not too long ago very few infants under 2,500 g survived, whereas now it is not uncommon for neonatologists to save kids who weigh in under 1 kg. So, if infant mortality were one of our endpoints, it may appear that women who work with VDTs have a *lower* infant mortality rate than the historical controls. Conversely, it may be expected that infants who are born weighing 800 g or less may have more abnormalities than kids who were born weighing 2,500 g or more. So, the overall prevalence of birth defects may be increasing over time. The result is that this outcome may look poor when compared with a historical control, irrespective of any effect VDTs may have. The lesson is that when a historical control is used, we have to be quite certain that nothing has changed in the interim that could affect its comparability with the group we are looking at now.

On rare occasions a control group may not be necessary at all. To quote Bradford Hill, "If we survey the deaths of infants in the first month of life and find that so many are caused by dropping the baby on its head on the kitchen floor I am not myself convinced that we need controls to satisfy us that this is a bad habit." The classic case of a study where a control group was unnecessary was the use of streptomycin for tuberculous meningitis; without treatment the disease was universally fatal, so that any improvement in survival was significant. Fortunately or unfortunately, such examples are rare.

SAMPLING

Needless to say the most accurate information about the incidence of adverse outcomes in pregnancy caused by working with VDTs would be gained if we could gather data from all women who had ever worked in front of these terminals at some point during their pregnancy. Just as obviously, however, this would be impractical; there may be hundreds of thousands of such women scattered over most of the globe. Practical considerations dictate that we could follow up only a small proportion of these women, and if we select them appropriately, our estimates won't be too far off. (However, the famous prediction in 1936 that Alf Landon would decisively beat FDR must serve as a constant reminder that "appropriately" isn't all that easy to define — much to Roosevelt's relief.) In this section we discuss various ways in which we could go about choosing the group or groups we will include in our study.

BASIC TERMINOLOGY

Population   All of the people to whom the results should be applicable constitute the populations. In this example the population would consist of all females who worked at VDTs at some time during their pregnancy (Fig. 2-3). (Note that "population" does not refer to all the people in the world; just to those who have a specific disorder, were exposed to some agent, or underwent some procedure.)

Figure 2-3   Population.

Sample   In most cases the population is quite large, and it is impractical to study all people. We limit our study to a subset of the population; this smaller group is called the sample (Fig. 2-4).

Cohort   Originally, cohort referred to a group of people born in the same year. Nowadays it has the broader, if less precise, meaning of a group of people who share some attribute. For instance, all people who began working at a specific job within a given time period can be referred to as a cohort, as can all people who entered the study at a certain time.

PROBABILITY SAMPLING

Probability sampling refers to a number of different strategies used to choose a sample. The term comes from the procedure used; every person in the population has a fixed and known probability of being selected to be part of the sample. For a number of reasons most studies try to use one or more of these strategies if at all possible.

The primary reason is that this method allows the investigator to generalize the results from the sample to the population, which is usually the major reason for doing a study. Second, it can tell the researcher the margin of error that could be expected from these estimates, that is, how far off the estimates can be. We see this in the reporting of polls, which often have a line stating that the results are accurate to within plus or minus 4 percent. In a related vein most statistical tests are based on the assumption of some sort of random sampling. When probability sampling is not used, we shouldn't use these tests (although that has never stopped people from doing so), and the ability to generalize the results from the sample to the population is questionable. (This is in contrast to the view of one politician who trusted letters he received more than polls and complained that the latter were "only" random.)

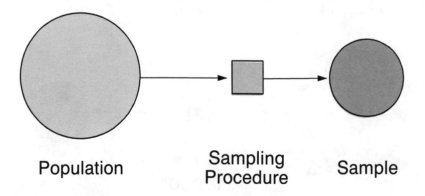

Population   Sampling Procedure   Sample

Figure 2-4   The sample is a subset of the population.

RANDOM SAMPLING

In **random sampling** (sometimes called "strictly random sampling" to differentiate it from the other varieties) each subject in the population has an equal chance of being chosen for the study. As we've mentioned, this approach maximizes the likelihood that the results of the study can be generalized to the entire population.

Random sampling is most often used in survey research (Fig. 2-5). Nearly all towns and cities have lists of taxpayers (for obvious reasons) or of street and house addresses. This makes it relatively simple for the researcher to select people, or at least dwellings, at random. These days about 98 percent of people have telephones, so it is also quite easy to draw a random sample from municipal or telephone lists, or from dialing digits at random.

Once we move out of the realm of surveys of the general population, however, it often becomes impossible to draw a pure random sample. We would have to know, for example, every company that used VDTs and all of the pregnant women at each business who had ever worked with VDTs in order to select people randomly for the study. More often we choose one or a number of businesses and hope that the use of VDTs within them is representative of companies in general, and that the women who work there are representative of female workers in other companies. We would then randomly select people within those companies for our study.

The same situation exists even for experimentally based studies. The hospital where a new treatment is tried out is not really chosen at random; it is most likely selected on the basis of convenience (e.g., the investigator works there or knows someone there who owes him a favor). The assumption is made that it is representative of hospitals in general, and that the randomly selected patients from that hospital are representative of the general population of patients with that condition. Unfortunately, these assumptions are not always correct and result in many of the various types of selection biases, which we discuss starting on p. 33 in *Threats to Validity.*

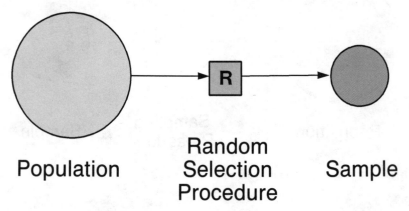

Population   Random   Sample
                    Selection
                    Procedure

Figure 2-5 Random sampling.

STRATIFIED RANDOM SAMPLING

There are some circumstances in which we may wish to deviate from strictly random sampling. One major reason is that, with random sampling, we may end up with too few people in one subgroup or another. For instance, if we thought that the teratogenicity of VDTs was related to the number of previous pregnancies, random sampling might result in very few women who had three or more children before working on the terminals; the sample would be too small to allow us to analyze the effects of parity. Similarly, we may want to have equal numbers of women in each age category to maximize the power of our statistical tests.

Conversely, we may want to ensure that our sample is equivalent to the general population in terms of a few key variables, such as age at first pregnancy or number of children (it's obviously not necessary to match for sex). Random sampling ensures this matching in the long run with large enough samples, but not necessarily in our particular study, especially if there are fewer than 1,000 subjects. By chance, we could over- or under-sample people from a particular age or parity group.

To achieve these goals, we divide the key variables into various levels, or **strata**. For instance, we can divide age into 10-year increments, or parity into one kid, two kids, and three or more (Fig. 2-6). Then subjects are selected randomly from the stratum into which they fall. If toward the end of the study we have enough women who have had one or two children, but not three or more, we would restrict entry into the study to only this latter group. Since we know how our strata deviate from a strictly random sample, we can correct for this during the analyses when we derive the prevalence figures.

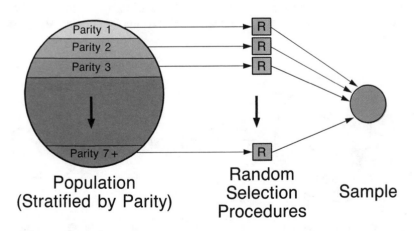

Population
(Stratified by Parity)

Random
Selection
Procedures

Sample

Figure 2-6   Stratified random samplings.

CLUSTER SAMPLING

In some designs it is impractical to assign individual subjects to the various groups. For example, in the Burlington Randomized Trial, nurse practitioners were placed in the offices of some family physicians to see whether they could reduce the cost of primary care without adversely affecting its quality. Outcome was measured at the level of the individual patient. However, since most families tend to use the same family doc, it would have been unfeasible to allocate randomly members of the same family to different practices. In this case each family was considered to be a **cluster**, and the unit of randomization was the family rather than the individual (Fig. 2-7).

However, the two, three, or more people in the same household cannot be considered to be independent of one another in terms of health status; they share the same diet, environment, and likely have similar attitudes toward exercise or other behaviors that affect health. Consequently, the husband's health is probably more correlated with his wife's than it is with that of another randomly chosen person.

Since the outcomes are correlated to some degree across people (who are usually considered to be independent in the usual statistical tests), studies that use cluster sampling usually need larger sample sizes than investigations in which the subjects are truly independent. How much larger the sample size has to be depends on the average number of people in the cluster, as well as on how strongly the variables are correlated within members of the cluster.

HAPHAZARD SAMPLING

In a **haphazard sample**, which is also called a "sample of convenience," subjects are selected on the basis of their availability, or in any other nonrandom way. For example, a researcher can interview people who pass

Population   Sampling
                     Procedure   Sample

Figure 2-7 Cluster sampling.

a certain street corner or take blood samples from the research assistants who work in his or her laboratory. There is always the very real danger that this is a biased, nonrepresentative sample. During the day, housewives, shift workers, or the unemployed are more likely to be walking around outside than are people who work 9 to 5, and the location of the specific corner may differentially favor people from one social class over another. (On Wall Street in New York and Bay Street in Toronto you were more likely to find Yuppies in 1986, and the unemployed in 1987.) Similarly, those working in a lab may be healthier, brighter, or disproportionately female compared with the population of interest.

Unfortunately, newscasters rely on just this sort of haphazard, "person in the street" interview to find out (often erroneously) what the people "really" think about some issue. Politicians, who rely on letters they receive, fall prey to the same trap; those who are concerned enough to write are not representative of the electorate in general. Lest we as researchers develop undue pride about our avoidance of such egregious errors as are committed by those who are untrained in the strict disciplines of science, two examples may suffice to remind us of our fallibility. Mueller and his colleagues developed a test for plasma unesterified fatty acid to be used for patients with neoplastic disease. Their 30 normal subjects were "members of the professional staff . . . or hospitalized normal volunteers." The sampling for this test may have been a marked improvement over another test, which studied hemolysate prothrombin consumption time; the authors gave no indication at all regarding how many normal blood samples were used, much less where they came from. To assume that these samples were randomly selected, and hence representative of normal people, requires a leap of faith that we, at least, cannot make.

SUBJECT ALLOCATION

As we have noted, in experimental studies, whether the person receives a treatment or some other intervention is under the control of the researcher. Just as subjects can be *selected* for the study in various ways, they can be assigned or **allocated** to the different groups in a number of ways.

Sometimes these two steps are combined; as subjects are selected from the population, they are assigned to groups. In other instances the two steps are explicitly differentiated; a sample is derived, and then a separate procedure is used to allocate the subjects to the various groups. However, it is important to be aware of these two steps because, many times, the first step (subject selection) is only implicit in the study. For example, while patients in a hospital can be randomly allocated to receive conventional therapy or a new treatment, there is actually an initial stage that may not have been acknowledged, namely, the selection of the hospitals where the study was carried out. In many instances this initial selection procedure was not random.

Unfortunately, the similarity of terms used to describe subject selection and allocation can lead to considerable confusion for the uninitiated or unwary reader, and offers an area of potential mischief for unscrupulous researchers (a group that fortunately does not include epidemiologists — often). In the above example the sample was randomly assigned to the treatment groups, but it was selected haphazardly. Describing the procedure as randomized, without adequately delineating the somewhat suspect origins of the sample, can be misleading.

RANDOMIZED ALLOCATION

With random allocation, all subjects in the sample have the same probability of being assigned to the experimental or to the control groups. (This is not the same as a specific subject having an equal probability of being assigned to the groups; for design reasons, one group may be deliberately larger than the other, so the probability of ending up in that group is higher. However, the probability would be the same for all subjects.) This ensures that in the long run (i.e., with a large number of subjects) any underlying factors that may affect the outcome are equivalent for each group.

The subjects are allocated to groups by a **randomization device** or **scheme**. If there are only two groups that are equal in size, this can be accomplished by a simple coin toss: if heads, then the first group, or if tails, the other group. However, it is more common to use a table of random numbers, which can be found in most introductory statistics books. These tables consist of many numbers, often listed in groups of five for the sake of readability, which are generated in a completely random fashion. An example of a small portion of a table of random numbers would look something like this:

92778	07201	92632	93521	18235
83855	98335	11980	90040	22843
85527	62908	55960	80310	46765
34606	20883	66096	23610	00765
37375	68228	49966	20361	57424
81839	59252	91022	94233	93928
67018	85005	03174	89887	94262

To assign subjects to two groups, the table is entered at random; if the first number is odd, for example, the subject is allocated to Group A, and if it is even, to Group B. The second subject is assigned in the same way on the basis of the next number in the table; "next" can mean moving your finger right, left, up, or down. When there are three groups, the subject is assigned to the first group if the number is 1, 2, or 3; to the second group if the number is 4, 5, or 6; and to the last group if the number is between 7 and 9. If a zero is encountered, it is simply ignored and the next nonzero number is used. Groups of unequal sizes can be created in the same way. If Group A is to be twice the size of B, then numbers 1 through 6 can be used to allot subjects to Group A, and 7 to 9 to Group B.

Now that you've mastered the arcane art of using tables of random numbers, the good news is that you probably won't need to do it, since most computers can produce random numbers quite easily. There are a number of programs that capitalize on this and produce lists of random assignments according to your specifications — equal numbers in all groups, one group twice the size of the others, and so on. However, they're based on the same principles as those of the random number table, so your mental effort was not in vain.

BLOCK RANDOMIZATION

Block randomization is a modification of random allocation, in which subjects are allocated in small blocks that usually consist of two to four times the number of groups (Fig. 2-8). If there are three groups, then the block size is often six, nine, or 12 subjects.

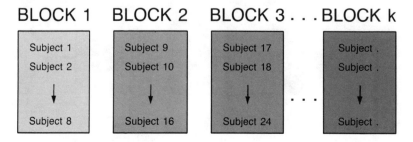

Figure 2-8 Allocation of subjects into blocks.

The subjects in the first block are randomly assigned so that there are equal numbers in each group (or, if the groups are not to be equal, they are assigned in proportion to the size of each group). The subjects in the succeeding blocks are then randomized in turn, until the final sample size is achieved (Fig. 2-9).

Block randomization ensures that, even if the study ends prematurely, there will be nearly equal numbers in all groups. With simple randomization it is possible to have a "run" of subjects assigned to one group; if the study ends at this point, an imbalance could result that would tend to reduce the efficiency of most statistical tests.

STRATIFIED ALLOCATION

The aim of **stratified allocation** is slightly different from that of stratified selection. In the selection phase stratification is used to ensure that the sample has certain desired characteristics. These characteristics may demand that the sample (1) matches the population on certain key variables, (2) includes sufficient numbers of subjects in all strata to permit subanalyses, or (3) has a normal distribution. The purpose of stratified allocations is more simple; it ensures that the groups do not differ too significantly on the stratification variables.

Stratified allocation is done when it is believed that the stratification variables may affect the outcome. If the groups are not balanced, any difference in outcome may result from these "nuisance" variables rather than from our intervention. For instance, if response to treatment is related to the patient's age, we do *not* want the experimental and control groups to differ on this factor.

For logistic reasons it is often impractical to have more than two or three stratifying variables, unless the available population is very large in relation to the sample size. Variables for stratification are chosen on the basis of their potential to affect the outcome. For example, since we felt that response to treatment was related to age but not to sex, only the former variable should be considered as a stratifying variable. If both age and duration of illness affect the outcome, but only one can be used as a stratification variable because of sample size limitations, the one that is more strongly associated with the outcome would be the variable to choose.

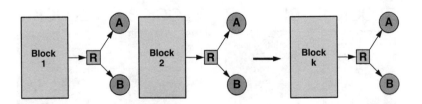

Figure 2-9   Block randomization.

MINIMIZATION

Minimization is a relatively recent and sophisticated method of assigning subjects to groups, and is used when there are many variables on which they should be matched. To keep matters simple, let's assume that we want to match the groups on only two variables: age and parity. The first few subjects are assigned to the groups by simple randomization. When a new person comes along, she is tentatively placed into each group in turn, and we compute what the mean age and parity level would be if she were in that group. The group to which she is ultimately assigned is based on minimizing the age and parity differences among the groups.

Because of the number of calculations required before a subject can be finally assigned (the number of variables multiplied by the number of groups), this method is unfeasible without a computer. Also, the criterion for "minimum differences between the groups" is somewhat arbitrary; how do we trade off an imbalance among the groups based on sex with differences based on age? For these reasons minimization is not yet widely used, although it may become more common in the future.

NONRANDOM (HAPHAZARD) ALLOCATION

Nonrandom allocation refers to situations in which subjects end up in the various groups by some manner other than having been randomly assigned. Let's assume that we wanted to compare the mean Apgar scores of kids whose mothers worked with VDTs against a group of kids whose mothers did not use display terminals. While we could *select* mothers at random from these two groups, the *allocation* would not have been random; they would have selected themselves to work or not work with the terminals.

The difficulty here is that there may be other factors on which these two groups of people differ. Some factors to be taken into consideration include the following:

1. Working women may be healthier than women in general (see the discussion on subject selection biases in *Threats to Validity*)
2. They may be working because they are poorer than other women (or become richer because they are working), and therefore provide a different prenatal environment
3. Even if we match for working status, those who have been chosen to be moved from typewriters to computers may be the brighter women.

In brief, the investigator has no control over factors that may, on the one hand, determine group membership and, on the other hand, affect the outcome.

The problem is even more acute in therapy trials. Clinical factors, which are also related to outcome, may have dictated whether the patient received medical or surgical treatment for his or her condition, or was given one drug rather than another. So, simply comparing the success rates of these haphazardly selected groups may lead to erroneous results, because we conclude that the difference between the groups was caused by the intervention rather than by the factors that originally placed the subject in one group rather than in the other.

MATCHING

The term **matching** can have two meanings: one applies at the level of the individual subject and the other describes the general strategy for selecting a control group.

Matching at the individual level means that a pair of experimental and control subjects are chosen to be as similar as possible in terms of certain key variables, such as age, sex, race, socioeconomic status, number of hospital admissions, or diagnosis. A person from the smaller subject pool is often chosen first (e.g., if there are fewer "exposed" than "nonexposed" people in a case-control design, the pool of potential experimental subjects is smaller than that of the controls). Then a subject from the other pool is selected and matched as closely as possible on the key characteristics. The larger the ratio of potential subjects to the desired number to be chosen, the more matching variables can be used. If there are not too many people to choose from, the number of matching variables must be reduced or the criteria for similarity are relaxed (e.g., matching for age within plus or minus 10 years rather than within 5). Matching results in the two groups being as similar as possible on these key variables.

At the level of the group, matching refers to selecting a control group that has certain characteristics as an aggregate. For example, subjects in this control group can be (1) patients at the same hospital, but with a different diagnosis; (2) drawn from the same community; or (3) working at similar jobs. Control subjects, however, are not matched to experimental subjects on a one-to-one basis.

The purpose of matching on certain variables is to eliminate the effect of those variables on group differences. If the two groups are matched on age, for example, any difference in outcome between the groups cannot result from this factor. The downside is that matching prevents us from examining at some later point the effect of age on the outcome. The moral is to match only when you're certain that you aren't ruling out examination of an association in which you may later be interested.

Groups are **undermatched** if they differ on some variable that is related to the outcome. The effect of undermatching is that group differences at the end may be caused by the variables that aren't matched. So, there is a fine line between overmatching, and thus being unable to explore potentially interesting relationships, and undermatching, which may cause your results to be explained by some extraneous variable.

THREATS TO VALIDITY

The purpose of any study is to tell us what is "really" happening in the world: Does streptokinase reduce cardiac mortality? What causes sudden infant death syndrome? Did the swine flu vaccination program do more good than harm? We hope that the results from our sample can be generalized to the population at large, so that our findings also hold true for similar people. Consequently it is disconcerting, at the least, to find different studies coming to opposite conclusions.

The major reason for these differences is that all studies have flaws involving (1) the definition of the disorder or phenomenon of interest, (2) the selection of the subjects, or (3) the design or execution of the study itself. Cook and Campbell call these flaws **threats to validity**. In this discussion we examine some of the more common ones, and see how they can affect the interpretation of the results. In *Measurement* we discuss those forms of bias that affect eliciting and recording information.

SUBJECT SELECTION BIASES

Subject selection biases involve a host of factors that may result in the subjects in the sample being unrepresentative of the population. We've already discussed one class of selection bias — nonrandom sampling. However, even with the best of sampling strategies, nature (human and otherwise) conspires against us in many ways. Sackett compiled a list of various biases, 57 at last count, and even this is probably incomplete. To keep life simple, we can think of two major types of subject selection biases: who gets *invited* to participate in a study, and who *accepts*. We cannot even attempt to provide a complete catalog of these two classes of factors; rather, the following three examples of invitational bias (healthy worker, incidence-prevalence, and Berkson's) and one of acceptance bias (volunteer) are illustrative only. We hope these examples help to enlighten and warn the reader of where things can go wrong.

HEALTHY WORKER BIAS

Randon sampling does not help us if the group from which the sample is drawn is unrepresentative of the population to which we want to generalize. For example, comparing the outcome of pregnancies of women who work with VDTs with those of a group of women chosen at random may open the researcher up to the **healthy worker** bias; that is, people who work are, as a group, healthier than the population as a whole. The entire adult population consists of those people who are working, those who are able to work but do not for one reason or another, and those who cannot work because of health problems. Any group of workers, by definition, does not include this last category of people that tends to lower the overall health status of the population. This selection bias operates even more strongly when the job applicants have to pass a physical examination, as in the Armed Forces or for certain labor-intensive occupations. Seltzer and Jablon, for example, found lower morbidity rates among people discharged from the Army than among people of similar ages in the general population. This effect was seen even 23 years after the men had been discharged. (Some have hypothesized that this is caused by Army food killing off the less fit before they can be discharged.)

The effects of this bias are to (1) make any sample drawn from a group of workers appear healthier than the general population; (2) make the standardized mortality rate (see *Measurement*) less than 1:1 when workers are compared with the general population; and (3) make the proportional mortality rate (see *Measurement*) for occupational hazards greater than 1.0 because of "borrowing" (i.e., if they are dying less from heart disease, they must be dying more from something else).

INCIDENCE-PREVALENCE (NEYMAN) BIAS

If a group is investigated a significant amount of time after the people have been exposed to a putative cause or after the disorder has developed, those who have died and those who have recovered will be missed. This is known as the **incidence-prevalence** bias or the **Neyman** bias. For example, a cross-sectional look at depressed patients in hospital misses those in whom the depression culminated in suicide or resolved itself. Similarly, a study of cardiac patients in a tertiary care hospital does not include (1) those who died before reaching hospital and (2) those whose myocardial infarction was not sufficiently severe to warrant transfer to a specialized facility.

As another example, even the latest version of the *Diagnostic and Statistical Manual of Mental Disorders* (1987) is somewhat pessimistic regarding the long-term prognosis in schizophrenia. However, this pessimism may be unwarranted, and may be based on the fact that most "natural history" studies use patients who are in hospital at a given time. Follow-up studies with patients who have been admitted for the first time, which are much less susceptible to the Neyman bias than cross-sectional ones, give a very different picture; according to these follow-up studies, the majority of patients — anywhere between 60 and 80 percent — go on to lead productive lives outside the hospital.

The effects of the Neyman bias can be in two different directions. Missing those who died before they could be included in the study makes the disorder look less severe, since the outcome is generally more positive than had all patients been included. Conversely, missing those who have already gotten better makes the outcome look grimmer. The net effect is often unknowable, and depends on the relative proportions of patients in the three groups (i.e., studied, died, and improved).

BERKSON'S BIAS

Berkson's bias is the spurious association found between some characteristic and a disease, and it results from admission rates to hospital (or any other setting where the study is carried out) being different for those persons (1) with the disease, (2) without the disease, and (3) with the characteristic. For example (Table 2-1), assume that in the general population there is no relationship at all between vaginal bleeding (the characteristic) and endometrial cancer (the disease).

Let us further assume that 10 percent of patients with endometrial cancer have vaginal bleeding and 10 percent of patients with other cancers have bleeding. If the probability of being admitted to hospital because of vaginal bleeding is 70 percent, if it's 10 percent because of endometrial cancer, and if it's 50 percent because of other forms of cancer, then:

1. Of the 100 patients with vaginal bleeding and endometrial cancer (cell A), 10 will be admitted because of endometrial cancer (i.e., 10 percent). Of the remaining 90 patients in cell A, 63 (70 percent) will be admitted because of vaginal bleeding, so that a total of 73 women will be admitted with endometrial cancer and bleeding.
2. Of the 100 patients with vaginal bleeding and other forms of cancer (cell B), 50 will be admitted because of the other cancers. Of the remaining 50, 35 (again, 70 percent) will be admitted because of vaginal bleeding, so that in total 85 will be admitted with bleeding and other cancers.
3. Of the 900 patients with endometrial cancer and no bleeding (cell C), 90 (again 10 percent) will be admitted because of endometrial cancer.

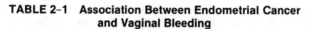

TABLE 2-1   **Association Between Endometrial Cancer and Vaginal Bleeding**

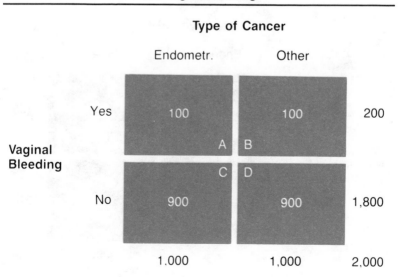

		Type of Cancer		
		Endometr.	Other	
Vaginal Bleeding	Yes	100 (A)	100 (B)	200
	No	900 (C)	900 (D)	1,800
		1,000	1,000	2,000

4. Of the 900 patients with other forms of cancer and no bleeding (cell D), 450 will be admitted because of the other cancers.

Table 2-2 shows the graphic results of these different admission rates. Now it appears that 44.8 percent of patients with endometrial cancer have vaginal bleeding, whereas only 15.9 percent of patients with other forms of cancer have vaginal bleeding. This apparent (and false) association is the result of different hospitalization rates for endometrial and other cancers and for vaginal bleeding. Thus, Berkson's bias comes into play whenever we sample from a setting in which there are different rates of admission for different disorders.

VOLUNTEER BIAS

To be ethical, most studies allow patients to refuse to participate. Thus the results are predicated to some degree on the assumption that those who do not volunteer are similar to those who do. However, there is now ample evidence to show that this is not the case and that volunteers differ systematically from nonvolunteers.

For example, the National Diet-Heart Study found that, compared with nonvolunteers, volunteers more frequently (1) were nonsmokers, (2) were concerned about health matters, (3) had a higher level of education, (4) were employed in professional and skilled jobs, (5) were Protestant or Jewish, (6) were living in households with children, and (7) were active in community affairs.

In one arm of the Coronary Drug Project the 5-year mortality rate for compliers (those who took 80 percent or more of their medication) was

TABLE 2-2   Results Caused by Different Hospitalization Rates for Characteristic (Bleeding) and Disease (Cancer)

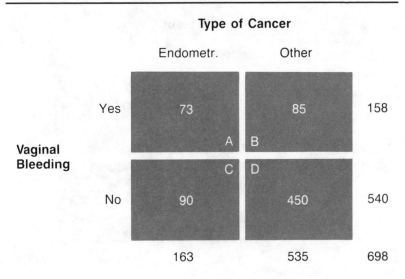

	Type of Cancer		
	Endometr.	Other	
Vaginal Bleeding — Yes	73 (A)	85 (B)	158
Vaginal Bleeding — No	90 (C)	450 (D)	540
	163	535	698

15.1 percent. It was almost twice as high among noncompliers (28.2 percent), even though the "medication" they were complying with was a placebo! Although all subjects were volunteers, those who complied with the treatment regimen were apparently a different breed from those who did not comply.

Even for those who participate in a trial, a type of volunteer bias may operate. The incidence of inactive tuberculosis was lower among volunteers who appeared early during a mass screening than among those who appeared later, whereas the opposite trend was noted for pneumoconiosis.

HAWTHORNE EFFECT

According to legend, worker productivity improved at the Hawthorne plant of the Western Electric Company not only when the illumination was increased, but also later when it was decreased. The reason for this was supposed to be the attention paid to the workers by the researchers and not the lighting itself. Although later studies showed that the increase in productivity likely resulted from other factors, the term **Hawthorne effect** has remained to explain the phenomenon that occurs when a subject's performance changes simply because he or she is being studied (some have referred to this as the psychological equivalent of the Heisenberg Uncertainty Principle).

For example, Frank reported that the introduction of a research project onto a hospital ward was "followed by considerable behavioral improvement in the patients," even though no medication or special treatments were involved. He felt that the most likely explanation was that "participation in the project raised the general level of interest of the treatment staff, and the patients responded favorably to this."

To counteract the Hawthorne effect it is often necessary to use an *attention control* group, which is treated exactly the same as the experimental group except for the active treatment. For example, studies of psychotherapy often employ a control group that meets with the therapist as frequently and for the same duration as does the treatment group, but the content of the session is not supposed to be therapeutic. In drug trials the control group receives a placebo, which usually involves taking the same number of pills at the same time of day as the experimental subjects.

BLINDING

One effect of the attention control group we just discussed is to **blind** the subject and perhaps the experimenter. A person is considered blind if he or she is unaware of the group to which a subject belongs. If only the subject is unaware but the experimenter knows, the study is called single blind. If both the subject and the researcher do not know, the study is labeled double blind. (Some people have proposed the term triple blind for the occasions when the subject and evaluator are blind, and the pharmacist has lost the key that tells who got the drug and who got the placebo. However, this is more a threat to the pharmacist's life than to validity.)

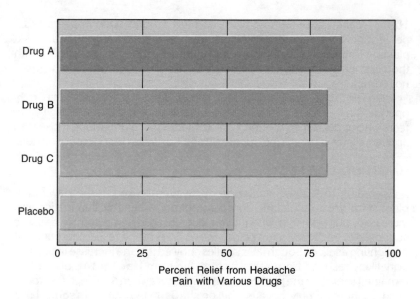

Figure 2-10 Results of this study show the placebo effect. In this case more than 50 percent of subjects on placebo experienced relief of headache pain.

The purpose of blinding is to prevent various biases from affecting the results. Subjects may show a *placebo effect* if they know they are receiving an active agent, or may not show it if they think they are not receiving the new drug. With single blinding, both groups should show an equivalent reaction. The magnitude of the placebo effect should not be underestimated (indeed, it's what kept medicine alive for a few millennia). The results of one typical study, shown in Figure 2-10, indicate that more than 50 percent of patients experienced relief of headache pain from placebos.

If the clinicians (or evaluators) were aware of group membership, they could be more alert or attentive to signs of improvement. Likewise, clinicians who know that a disease should be present may be more diligent when looking for it (*diagnostic suspicion bias*). Rosenthal conducted a series of studies that showed that what a researcher expects to find in an experiment affects what does occur, irrespective of whether the subjects are humans or rats.

CONFOUNDING

Confounding is the illusory association between two variables when in fact no such association exists. It is caused by a third variable (the "confounder"), which is correlated with the first two. For example, Table 2-3 shows bifocal use (needed or not) and nocturnal enuresis (present or absent) in a group of 200 patients.

**TABLE 2-3   Relationship Between the Need for Bifocals
and Nocturnal Enuresis**

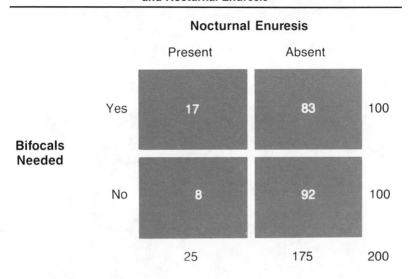

The odds ratio is 1.93, which indicates that persons who need bifocals are twice as likely to have enuresis as those who don't need bifocals. (This may be related to the supposed link between masturbation and blindness.)

However, a closer look at these data shows that there are actually two age groups involved (Table 2-4). For each age group there is no association between bifocal use and enuresis. In those under age 60, 5 percent of bifocal users are enuretic (1 of 20 subjects), as are 5 percent of nonusers (4 of 80 subjects). For those over age 60, 20 percent are enuretic, irrespective of bifocal use. The confounder here is age; bifocal users are more apt to be over age 60, which is also the group that has the higher rate of enuresis. (Fig. 2-11)

**TABLE 2-4   No Association Between Bifocal Need and Nocturnal Enuresis
When Subjects are Divided by Age**

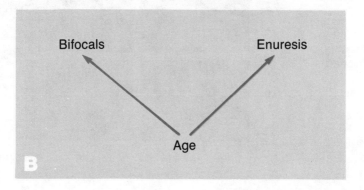

Figure 2-11 A, When unaware of the confounder, it appears that there is a direct association between enuresis and bifocals. B, There is a direct association between age (confounder) and bifocals and between age and enuresis.

CONTAMINATION

In studies in which one group receives the experimental treatment and another group gets either conventional treatment or a placebo, the validity of the results is predicated on the *purity* of the groups. If some subjects in the control group receive the new treatment, both groups will improve to some degree (assuming that the treatment works). Thus, differences between the groups are diminished or even eliminated. This condition is referred to as **contamination**.

Contamination is a particular problem when a medication used in a study is also available over the counter or as an ingredient in other compounds (e.g., aspirin), or when it can be prescribed by family physicians who are unaware (or have forgotten) that certain drugs should not be given to some of their patients. However, contamination is not limited to drug trials; it can occur with any form of intervention, such as respite care for those taking care of demented elderly, psychotherapy, and similar maneuvers in which subjects in the control group receive some form of the treatment.

In cohort and case-control studies contamination is caused by misclassification, that is, assigning exposed subjects to the nonexposed group or vice versa. This is often caused by errors in recall by the subjects.

The effect of contamination is to reduce differences between the treated and untreated groups. This may lead us to draw the erroneous conclusion that the intervention is of limited or no use.

COINTERVENTION

Cointervention refers to subjects in a study receiving therapies other than those given as part of the experiment that affect the outcome of interest. For example, some subjects in a study that compares the effectiveness of various nonsteroidal anti-inflammatory drugs for arthritis could be given other drugs by another physician, be enrolled in a program using transcutaneous stimulation, or might be taking over-the-counter aspirin.

Cointervention differs from contamination in two ways: (1) the intervention and (2) the groups that are affected. First, contamination refers to the control group receiving the experimental intervention, whereas cointervention refers to some treatment other than the one under investigation. Second, all groups in a study can be witting or unwitting recipients of a certain cointervention, but only the control group can be contaminated.

Although all groups can be subject to cointervention, it is a particular danger when the control subjects do not improve or even deteriorate on placebo. If any other clinician is involved in the case and unaware of the study, he or she may prescribe other treatments to help the person, thereby minimizing differences between the groups. If subjects in all groups receive other therapies, then it becomes almost impossible to determine if the results are caused by the treatment under study, by the cointervention, or by both.

REGRESSION TOWARD THE MEAN

Regression toward the mean refers to the phenomenon whereby groups of subjects that are chosen because of their extreme score on any variable will have scores that are less extreme and closer to the mean value when they are retested. The reason is that any test result we observe — some serum value, a decision based on an x-ray, or a score on a paper and pencil test — is comprised of two parts: the *true* score and an *error* score. Written out in the form of an equation, we say:

Observed Score = True Score ± Error Component

There are many sources of error (see the discussion in *Measurement with Continuous Variables* on reliability), including variations in the machine, biologic variation within the subject, motivation, fatigue, and recording error. The assumption is that this error component is random, sometimes adding to the true score and sometimes diminishing it. We can never see the true score, only the observed score.

When we select a group because of its extreme scores (either very high or very low), we are including two types of persons: (1) those whose true scores are extreme and (2) those whose true scores do *not* fall in the extreme range, but the error component added to the true score has placed them in the extreme region. Similarly, we have excluded persons whose true scores are extreme, but whose observed scores are below the cut-off level. For example, let's assume that we're using a test with a mean of 50, and a score of 70 or above identifies the most extreme 2 percent of the sample, which is the group we want to include in our study. We've shown the true score plus or minus the error component for the 10 subjects whose observed scores are over 70 and for a few of the other subjects (Fig. 2-12). Thus we have biased our sample to include an overrepresentation of people who have error scores in the direction *away from* the mean. Since the error component is random, when these people are retested only half of them will have error scores away from the mean (keeping them in the extreme range), and half will have error scores that move the observed score closer to the mean. On the whole, the group average on the second testing will be closer to the mean than on the first testing.

In practical terms this means that if we select a group of subjects because they appear abnormal on some test (that is, their score differs from the mean) and do *nothing* to them, they will seem to improve (move closer to the mean) when they are retested. So, if we had intervened, it would be impossible to know if the improvement was caused by us or simply by regression effects.

The magnitude of this effect is inversely related to the reliability of the test; the less reliable the test is, the greater the regression effect. The reason is that reliability expresses the relative contributions of the true score and the error scores, so that an unreliable test has a large error component (see the discussion on reliability in *Measurement with Continuous Variables* for more detail).

Regression toward the mean can be minimized in two ways: (1) by increasing the reliability of the test, and (2) by testing each subject at least twice and requiring all the tests to be extreme before he or she is included in the study. This is often done in hypertension trials in which the person has to have three consecutive abnormal readings before being called hypertensive.

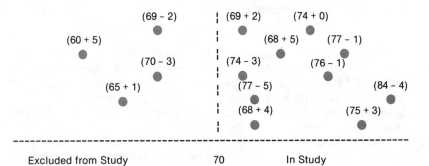

Figure 2-12 True score ± error component for 10 subjects with observed scores over 70, and four subjects with observed scores under 70.

COHORT EFFECTS

Nowadays a **cohort** refers to a group of people chosen because they share some common characteristic (e.g., employment in a specific job, or exposure to a given agent). Previously, however, cohort was used in a narrower sense and meant a group of similar age, the members of which having in common only their year of birth. Cohorts of this type have been extremely useful in elucidating many epidemiologic findings, such as increases in longevity and height over time. A danger arises when one attempts to attribute a *causal* factor to differences among age cohorts, since one cohort differs from another on many variables other than age.

For example, studies done in the 1940s and 1950s tended to show a decline in intelligence over the age of 50 by comparing various age cohorts on a standardized test. Subsequently longitudinal studies have demonstrated that, while performance on timed tasks does decrease, scores on other tests either remain stable or actually increase with age (we can all now breathe a sigh of relief). The problem with the original studies was that not only were the older subjects more advanced in years than the younger ones, they were also exposed to a very different educational and cultural environment, which accounted for most of the differences among the cohorts and hence for most of the apparent decline.

ECOLOGIC FALLACY

Ecologic studies attempt to demonstrate a relationship between two variables, such as suicide rate and religion, by using aggregate data. These are data about groups of people rather than individuals. For example, we can look at the rates of lung cancer per 100,000 individuals in a number of cities, and see if these are correlated with pollution levels.

While this technique is very inexpensive and has at times led to useful findings, there is one major problem — there is no guarantee that those people who developed lung cancer were the same ones who were exposed to the pollution. That is, it is possible (although unlikely) that pollution is unrelated to cancer of the lung, but that pollution is caused by large factories. We know that cigarette smoking is related to social class, and that factory workers smoke more heavily than the general population. So, it may be that pollution is simply a marker for heavy smoking, and it is the smoking that is producing cancer.

The ecologic fallacy was nicely demonstrated by Robinson, who showed that there was a strong relationship ($r=0.62$) between literacy rates and the proportion of non-native born people; that is, regions with the largest number of immigrants had the lowest rates of illiteracy. Since most immigrants had relatively little education, especially in the 1930s when the data were collected, this seems to fly in the face of common sense. However, the individual correlation between literacy and foreign birth was -0.12, which is lower in magnitude (correlations based on individuals are almost always lower than ecologic correlations) and in the reverse direction.

The explanation is that immigrants usually settle in large cities, which have high rates of literacy, rather than in rural areas where literacy rates are lower. Thus, *areas* with low rates of illiteracy have a high proportion of immigrants, but illiteracy and immigrant status are correlated (albeit weakly) within the *individual*.

EPIDEMIOLOGIC RESEARCH STRATEGIES

The hallmark of a scientific theory is that its hypotheses are capable of being disproved. This does not always require experiments under the control of the researcher; astronomers haven't yet figured out how to experimentally induce stars to form or evolve. However, when experimental studies can be done, they can provide powerful tests of hypotheses that are not feasible when we have to rely solely on observations of naturally occurring events.

Over the years many different study designs have been developed to deal with the multitude of research questions that have been asked. We cannot begin to describe all of these methods here; entire books have been written on just this one area. Rather we have chosen the six designs that are used most frequently. The first four (cross-sectional, ecologic, cohort, and case-control) are commonly referred to as **descriptive** or **analytic** designs. These are most appropriate when, for one reason or another, experimental control over the independent variable is not feasible. This would include, for instance, exposure to potentially harmful agents (e.g., cigarette smoke), situations in which there may be a long interval between exposure and outcome (such as diethylstilbestrol use and vaginal cancer in female offspring), or when our state of knowledge (or rather, ignorance) doesn't yet allow us to state whether there is an effect that's worth following up with a more expensive trial.

The last two designs (randomized control trial and cross-over) are called **experimental**, since the intervention is under the control of the researcher. These methods are used (or should be used) in therapy trials, since their results are least susceptible to the various threats to validity.

The important point is that the choice of study design depends on the question being asked. Usually several methods are possible, and we may look for the strongest (i.e., the one that allows the fewest alternative explanations for the results). However, we may instead opt for a "quick and dirty" design, even if it isn't the optimal one, simply to see if there is anything worth looking into at greater expense.

NOMENCLATURE

Table 2-5 is based on the nomenclature introduced by Kleinbaum, Kupper, and Morgenstern and modified by the Department of Clinical Epidemiology and Biostatistics at McMaster University.

TABLE 2-5   Nomenclature for Epidemiologic Research Strategies

	Subject Allocation
N	Pool of eligible subjects
R	Random assignment
R	Stratified random assignment
	Intervention
E	Exposure to intervention or causal factor
$\bar{E}$	Nonexposure
T	Treatment
$\bar{T}$	No treatment
	Outcome
--| 1 yr |--	Follow-up (1 year)
C	Prevalent case
$\bar{C}$	Noncase
D	Outcome present; incident case; or death
$\bar{D}$	Outcome not present; noncase; or survivor
O	A continuous outcome

DESCRIPTIVE AND ANALYTIC STRATEGIES
CROSS-SECTIONAL SURVEY
Design

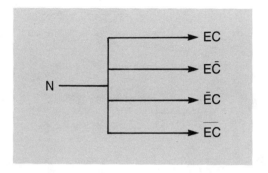

Example
A group of women (N) are interviewed to determine (1) their use of video display terminals (E) and (2) whether they had a miscarriage (C).

Major Features
Exposure and caseness are determined simultaneously.

Advantages
1. This design is relatively inexpensive and simple to carry out because no follow-up is required.
2. No one is exposed to the putative causal agent because of the study, or denied a potentially beneficial therapy.

Disadvantages
1. A cross-sectional design can establish association, but it is impossible to determine causation, since exposure and caseness are determined at the same time.
2. It is impossible to ensure that confounders are equally distributed among the groups.
3. Often either exposure or caseness or both depend upon recall, which is fallible.
4. This design is susceptible to the Neyman bias, that is, cases with early deaths and those in which evidence of exposure has disappeared are missed.
5. The groups could end up having very different sample sizes, resulting in a loss of statistical efficiency.

ECOLOGIC STUDY

Design

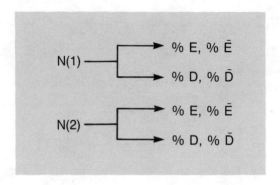

Example

Ecologic studies are used quite often in cancer research, in which the rates of cancer of different organs are examined by geographic area (county, province, or state). This has led to some fruitful hypotheses regarding the association between cancer of the esophagus and diet in Eastern Europe and China, for instance.

Major Features

The group, usually defined geographically, is the unit of analysis, and the data are most often already available.

Advantages

1. Data are usually available, so this type of study is quite inexpensive.

Disadvantages

1. We know how many people were exposed within each group and how many have the outcome, but *not* how many exposed people have the outcome. That is, it is quite possible that the outcome occurred in unexposed people and the variables are not related (see the discussion in *Threats to Validity* on ecologic fallacy).
2. Correlations from ecologic studies are usually much higher than in studies where both variables are gathered on the same individuals.

COHORT STUDY

Design

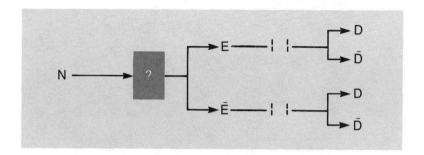

Example

A group of women who used VDTs during their pregnancy and a second group who did not use them are followed to determine the rates of miscarriages, stillbirths, and congenital abnormalities.

Major Features

Exposure to the putative causal agent or treatment is *not* under the researcher's control. Subjects are divided into exposed (or treated) and nonexposed (or untreated) groups on the basis of past history. The design can be prospective (following the groups forward in time from the present), or retrospective (choosing groups that were formed some time in the past, and then following them forward from that time to the present).

Advantages

1. Treatment is not withheld from subjects and they are not artificially subjected to potential hazards.
2. Subjects can be matched for possible confounders.
3. When the design is prospective, eligibility criteria and outcome assessments can be standardized.
4. It is administratively easier and less costly than an RCT.
5. It can establish the timing and directionality of events.

Disadvantages

1. It may be difficult to obtain controls if therapy is popular or if most people have been exposed.
2. Exposure may be related to some other unknown factor that is correlated with the outcome (confounding).
3. Blindness among subjects and assessors may be difficult to achieve.
4. It is expensive to do well.
5. It may violate some statistical tests based on the assumption of randomization.
6. For rare disorders, large sample sizes or follow-up periods are necessary.

CASE-CONTROL STUDY

Design

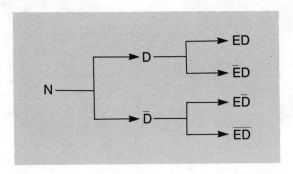

Example

The mothers of children born with (D) and without (D̄) birth defects are interviewed to determine whether or not they used video display terminals during their pregnancy.

Major Features

The groups are identified on the basis of the *outcome* (e.g., birth defects), and the search for exposure (to video display terminals) is retrospective.

Advantages

1. It can be done relatively quickly and inexpensively.
2. It may be the only feasible method for very rare disorders, or for situations in which there is a long lag between exposure and outcome.
3. It usually requires fewer subjects than cross-sectional studies.

Disadvantages

1. It relies on recall or records to determine exposure, and both are notoriously inaccurate.
2. The groups may be confounded, that is, exposure may have been caused by some other factor that is correlated with the outcome (e.g., income, area of residence, age).
3. It may be difficult to select and then find an appropriate control group.
4. If the index group is aware of the hypothesis, there is the possibility of recall bias.

EXPERIMENTAL DESIGNS

RANDOMIZED CONTROLLED TRIAL

Design

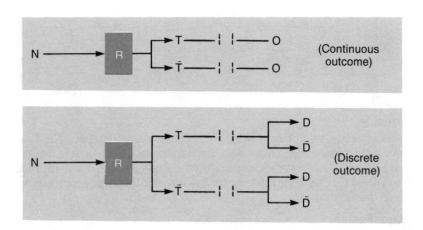

(Continuous outcome)

(Discrete outcome)

Example

Hemiplegic stroke patients currently receiving physiotherapy are randomly assigned to receive or not receive transcutaneous stimulation. After 3 months, they are compared on walking speed (continuous outcome) and presence or absence of footdrop (discrete outcome).

Major Features

Subject allocation to treatments or exposure is under the control of the experimenter.

Advantages

1. Groups are likely more comparable because confounding variables are probably balanced.
2. There is a greater likelihood that patients, staff, and assessors can be blinded.
3. Most statistical tests rest on the assumption of random allocation.

Disadvantages

1. These trials are expensive in terms of time and money.
2. Those who volunteer may not be representative of all patients.
3. A potentially effective treatment is withheld from some subjects, or some may be exposed to a possibly dangerous one.

CROSS-OVER DESIGN

Design

Example

Patients are randomly allocated to receive carbamazepine (CBZ) to control their manic-depressive disorder or a placebo. After 4 weeks they are given a placebo until all the drug is out of their system. Then those who had been given CBZ are given placebo for 4 weeks, and those given placebo are given the active drug.

Major Features

Randomization is under the researcher's control; all patients receive both the active treatment and the placebo (or control treatment).

Advantages

1. Subjects serve as their own controls, thereby reducing error variance. Consequently, fewer subjects generally are needed than for RCTs.
2. All subjects receive the treatment at least for some period.
3. Statistical tests assuming randomization can be used.
4. Blindness of patients, staff, and assessors can be maintained.

Disadvantages

1. Subjects who responded to the treatment are taken off it and given placebo (or the alternative treatment).
2. The wash-out period with some drugs can be quite lengthy, during which time the patients are often given placebos.
3. It cannot be used if the treatment has any permanent effects (e.g., educational programs, physiotherapy, behavior therapy).

C.R.A.P. DETECTORS

C.R.A.P. DETECTOR II-1

Question   In one of the seminal books on the etiology of homosexuality Bieber and his associates derived their sample by mailing three copies of a questionnaire to fellow members of a New York-based psychoanalytic society. The analysts filled them out for any homosexual patients they had in therapy. If the psychiatrist had fewer than three such patients in treatment, he or she was to fill out the remaining questionnaires on male heterosexual patients; the heterosexual subjects constituted the control group. What are the problems with this sampling strategy?

Answer   Unfortunately a listing of all the problems would fill a book thicker than this one. First, persons who elect to go into psychoanalysis are not representative of the general population. Obviously, those who are happy with their lives never spend time on the analytic couch. Second, those who are unhappy but poor must settle for less comfortable and less expensive chairs, or get no help at all. Finally, leaving the choice of which patients to include up to the individual analysts opens the door to a host of biases; it is doubtful whether the sample would include patients who didn't improve or who didn't match the psychoanalytic sample.

C.R.A.P. DETECTOR II-2

Question   Those who disapprove of social assistance programs state that welfare fosters dependence, and encourages people to behave in ways that enable them to remain on assistance for a long time. The opponents buttress their arguments with surveys showing that, at any one time, the majority of welfare recipients have been on it for extended periods. How much can we trust these data?

Answer   This is a nice example of the incidence-prevalence bias. Figure 2-13A shows the proportion of women who have ever received Aid for Families with Dependent Children (AFDC), and how long they were on it. Of these women, 30 percent were on AFDC for only 1 or 2 years, and 70 percent received it for less than 8 years. However, if the investigators had done a cross-sectional survey that asked women currently on AFDC how long they had been on it, a very different picture would emerge. Now, as Figure 2-13B shows, the vast majority (65 percent) have been getting benefits for more than 7 years. The problem is that long-term recipients are more likely to be picked up in a one-time survey than short-term recipients who had been on AFDC in the past, but were not at the time of the survey.

Percent of Women Ever on AFDC

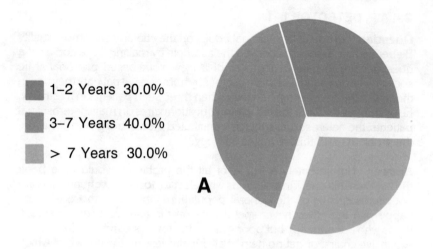

Percent of Women on AFDC at a Particular Time

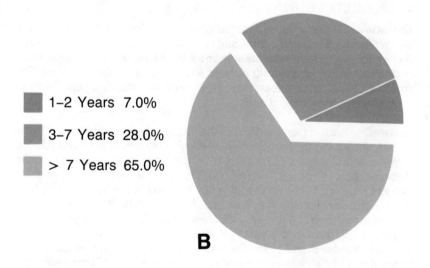

Figure 2-13 *A*, Percentage of women who have ever received AFDC and length of time they received it. *B*, Percentage of women who received AFDC at a particular time and the length of time they had been receiving it.

C.R.A.P. DETECTOR II-3

Question Schroeder, among others, concluded that there was a relationship between water hardness and cardiovascular disease. Specifically, he found a correlation of -0.56, which indicated that states with the softest water had the highest death rates for heart disease. Should you be worried if you live in an area with soft water?

Answer Schroeder's study used data aggregated at the level of states, and as such it was susceptible to the ecologic fallacy. Comstock followed up this finding by gathering data on individuals, and found no relationship between cardiovascular disease and trace elements in water. So, what holds at the level of the community or state may not obtain for the individual.

C.R.A.P. DETECTOR II-4

Question According to Ederer the 10 top batters in the American League in 1968 had a mean batting average of .414, and the 10 worst batted an average of .083, in the first week of play. As can be seen in Figure 2-14, by the second week both groups were batting in the low .200s. Does this mean that the good batters suddenly got worse, and the bad batters mysteriously got better?

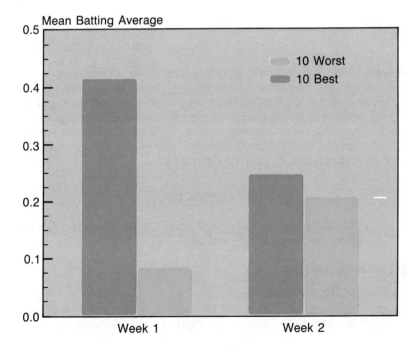

Figure 2-14 Mean batting average of 10 best and 10 worst batters.

Figure 2-15 Example of regression toward the mean effect: the higher the baseline serum cholesterol level, the greater the subsequent improvement, regardless of diet.

Answer   This is an example of the regression toward the mean effect; on the average, persons chosen because they are above the mean on one occasion tend to "regress" down toward it at a second measurement period, and those below the mean regress upward. Ederer showed the same effect with serum cholesterol (Fig. 2-15): the higher the baseline level, the greater the later "improvement," whether the subjects had been on a cholesterol-lowering diet or a control diet.

REFERENCES

Chenier NM. Reproductive hazards at work. Ottawa: Canadian Advisory Council on the Status of Women, 1982.

DESIGN ELEMENTS

Number of Observations

Bagby RM, Silverman I, Ryan DP, Dickens SE. Effects of mental health legislative reforms in Ontario. Can Psychol 1987; 28:21-29.

Comparison Groups

Hill AB. Statistical methods in clinical and preventive medicine. Edinburgh: Livingstone, 1962:365.

Hinshaw HC, Feldman WH, Pfuetze KH. Treatment of tuberculosis with streptomycin: summary of observations on 100 cases. JAMA 1946; 132:778-782.

SAMPLING

Cluster Sampling

Donner A, Birkett N, Buck C. Randomization by cluster: sample size requirements and analysis. Am J Epidemiol 1981; 114:906-914.

Spitzer WO, Sackett DL, Sibley JC, Roberts RS, Gent M, Kergin DJ, Hackett BC, Olynich A. The Burlington Randomized Trial of the nurse practitioner. N Engl J Med 1974; 290:251-256.

Haphazard Sampling

Mueller PS, Watkin DM. Plasma unesterified fatty acid concentrations in neoplastic disease. J Lab Clin Med 1961; 57:95-108.

Quick AJ. Hemolysate prothrombin consumption time: a new test for thromboplastinogenic coagulation defects. J Lab Clin Med 1961; 57:290-299.

THREATS TO VALIDITY

Cook, TD, Campbell DT. Quasi-experimentation: design issues for field settings. Chicago: Rand McNally, 1979.

Subject Selection Biases

Sackett DL. Bias in analytic research. J Chronic Dis 1979; 32:51-63.

Healthy Worker Bias

Seltzer CC, Jablon S. Effects of selection on mortality. Am J Epidemiol 1974; 100:367-372.

Incidence-Prevalence Bias

American Psychiatric Association. Diagnostic and statistical manual of mental disorders. 3rd ed. revised. Washington: APA, 1987.

Harding CM, Zubin J, Strauss JS. Chronicity in schizophrenia: fact, partial fact, or artifact? Hosp Community Psychiatry 1987; 38:477-486.

Volunteer Bias

American Heart Association. The National Diet-Heart Study: final report. American Heart Association Monograph No. 18. New York: AHA, 1980.

Cochrane AL. The application of scientific methods to industrial and social medicine. In: Morris JN, ed. Uses of epidemiology. Baltimore: Williams & Wilkins, 1964.

Coronary Drug Project Research Group. Influence of adherence to treatment and response to cholesterol on mortality in the Coronary Drug
Project. N Engl J Med 1980; 303:1038-1041.

Hawthorne Effect

Bramel D, Friend R. Hawthorne, the myth of the docile worker, and class
bias in psychology. Am Psychol 1981; 36:867-878.
Frank JD. Persuasion and healing. Baltimore: Johns Hopkins Press, 1961.
Parsons HM. What happened at Hawthorne? Science 1974; 183:922-932.

Blinding

Beecher HK. The powerful placebo. JAMA 1955; 159:1602-1606.
Rosenthal R. Experimenter effects in behavioral research. New York:
Appleton-Century-Crofts, 1966.

Cohort Effects

Horn JL, Donaldson G. On the myth of intellectual decline in adulthood. Am
Psychol 1976; 31:701-719.

Ecologic Fallacy

Robinson WS. Ecological correlations and the behavior of individuals. Am
Sociol Rev 1950; 15:351-357.

EPIDEMIOLOGIC RESEARCH STRATEGIES

Nomenclature

Kleinbaum DG, Kupper LL, Morgenstern H. Epidemiologic research: principles and quantitative methods. Belmont, CA: Lifetime Learning Publications, 1982.

C.R.A.P. DETECTORS

Bieber I, Dain HJ, Dince PR, et al. Homosexuality. New York: Basic Books,
1962.
Comstock GW. Fatal arteriosclerotic heart disease, water hardness at
home, and socioeconomic characteristics. Am J Epidemiol 1971;
94:1-10.
Duncan GJ, Hill MS, Hoffman SD. Welfare dependence within and across
generations. Science 1988; 239:467-471.
Ederer F. Serum cholesterol changes: effects of diet and regression toward
the mean. J Chronic Dis 1972; 25: 277-289.
Schroeder HA. Relationship between mortality from cardiovascular disease
and treated water supplies: variations in states and 163 largest munici-
palities of the United States. JAMA 1960; 172:1902-1908.

TO READ FURTHER

SAMPLING

Abramson JH. Survey methods in community medicine. Edinburgh: Churchill-Livingstone, 1974.

Levy P, Lemeshow S. Sampling for health professionals. Belmont, CA: Lifetime Learning Publications, 1980.

THREATS TO VALIDITY

Ederer F. Patient bias, investigator bias and the double-masked procedure in clinical trials. Am J Med 1975; 58:295-299.

Morgenstern H. Uses of ecologic analysis in epidemiological research. Am J Public Health 1982; 72:1336-1344.

Rosenthal R, Rosnow RL. The volunteer subject. New York: Wiley, 1975.

Sackett DL. Bias in analytic research. J Chronic Dis 1979; 32:51-63.

Walter SD. Cause-deleted proportional mortality analysis and the healthy worker effect. Stat Med 1986; 5:61-71.

EPIDEMIOLOGIC RESEARCH STRATEGIES

Cook TD, Campbell DT. Quasi-experimentation: design issues for field settings. Chicago: Rand McNally, 1979.

Kleinbaum DG, Kupper LL, Morgenstern H. Epidemiologic research: principles and quantitative methods. Belmont, CA: Lifetime Learning Publications, 1982.

MEASUREMENT

We live in a cancerophobic society. For several decades the man on the street has been bombarded with the carcinogen of the week to the point of numbing exhaustion. This epidemic reached ludicrous limits when it was announced, in all seriousness, that mother's milk "caused" cancer because it contained trace amounts of PCBs and other awful chemicals, and that children should be breast-fed for a maximum of 6 months.

In part, the present dilemma can be laid at the feet of zealous legislators and news-hungry media folks; in part, the problem exists simply because our technical expertise has far outstripped our legislative apparatus. Laws about cancer in the environment were passed several decades ago, when the prevailing attitude was that any amount of a carcinogen in the soil, air, or water was too much. Since that time, technical improvements in analytic instrumentation have allowed us to detect trace amounts of chemicals that are orders of magnitude smaller than the amounts detectable when the laws were passed (literally equivalent to a martini made with a drop of vermouth in a swimming pool of gin). However, the laws remain on the books and any attempt to repeal them at this stage would promote a rapid demise to any political career.

In part, too, the issue is epidemiologic. Epidemiologists, oncologists, and toxicologists tend to view the issue of causation as a binary variable — either something causes cancer or it doesn't. Admittedly, some attempt is made to quantify the risk by extrapolation from animal data to humans. Nevertheless, it would certainly assist the field, and perhaps our quality of life, if we would pause to ask just how much cancer a particular agent might cause. Of course, this question demands some means of quantifying the degree of risk to life and limb from a particular agent.

This chapter deals explicitly with this issue, discussing a variety of **measures of association** used by epidemiologists. The problems to which these measures can be applied are far ranging, from the estimation of the risk to health from an environmental agent, to the benefit of treatment, to the agreement between a diagnostic test and a "gold standard," and to issues of observer agreement.

ISSUES IN CHOOSING A MEASURE

The issue of measurement is critical to much of science. Lord Kelvin, a distinguished physicist of the 1800s, once said

> I often say that when you can measure what you are speaking about, and express it in numbers, you know something about it; but when you cannot express it in numbers, your knowledge is of a meager and unsatisfactory kind; it may be the beginning of knowledge, but you have scarcely, in your thoughts, advanced to the stage of science whatever the matter may be.

Epidemiology is not immune to these admonitions. The issue of measurement in many sciences is, by and large, a technical issue of instrumentation, and of developing the right bit of apparatus to measure some phenomenon with the appropriate degree of precision. In epidemiology the issues are a bit more conceptual, and much thought must be directed to the appropriate selection of which variable to measure in the first place. Often the choice of variable represents a deliberate compromise; for example, in looking at the effects of an educational strategy for practicing physicians one could decide to measure the increase in knowledge of the participants, a variable that is likely sensitive to the educational strategy and can be easily tested with methods like multiple choice questions. Unfortunately, this choice begs the issue of whether the increased knowledge will be translated into a change in physician behavior with patients. In turn, we should worry whether the doctor's admonitions will change patient behavior, whether this behavior change will actually result in improved health, and whether the improvement in health will result in increased longevity or decreased morbidity. It is evident that the further we get from the intervention, the more socially relevant the outcomes are, but the less likely they are to be sensitive to the intervention.

THE DIMENSIONS OF MEASUREMENT

Epidemiologists have categorized the wide number of potential choices in the measurement of the effects of illness into the six Ds — death, disease, disability, discomfort, dissatisfaction, and debt. A little creativity can easily result in some additions to the list: psychiatrists would like to look at dysphoria and depression, and sociologists might examine disenfranchisement or dysfunction.

Some of these variables, like death and debt, are relatively easy to measure, and hence are frequently used in studies in epidemiology. Others, like dissatisfaction and disability, are notoriously difficult to measure, and have been the making of many a career in epidemiology. We will avoid, for the most part, the technical issues surrounding the measurement of these variables; the important point is that the Ds serve as a reminder that measurement of dependent variables or outcomes need not be confined to the traditional measures like death and disease.

The choice of an outcome variable is almost inevitably a compromise based on the interplay among the several following factors:

1. **Precision of Measurement.** Measures that are subject to a large degree of random variation or individual interpretation are less useful than measures that are more precise. The judgment of precision cannot be made on an a priori basis; careful studies have shown appallingly high error rates in many areas of clinical medicine, such as radiology, that conventional wisdom would suggest are highly objective. Methods to assess precision are reviewed later in this section.

2. **Logistical Factors.** Measures are often chosen simply because they are inexpensive. Cost is certainly one criterion, as are other logistical factors like the likelihood of obtaining compliance, or the ease of entering the data.

3. **Ethical Issues.** Some measurements are unsuitable for ethical reasons. No ethics committee would permit coronary angiography to be performed on all patients in a trial, regardless of cost, simply because of the risks associated with the procedure (unless the test was a part of the patients' regular care).

4. **Importance.** Often the most important variables, in terms of their burden on the affected individual, are the most impractical to use in studies. One good example is death. It has considerable importance to the individuals involved. However, although it is precise and easy to measure, death is often rejected as an outcome variable in studies because it occurs too infrequently (thank goodness), and thus the follow-up period required would be too long. As a result, investigators often substitute other variables that are less important, but more available for measurement. As one example, hypoglycemic agents were adopted because they demonstrated the appropriate effect on blood sugar, which is much easier to measure than diabetes (although not as relevant). Much later the widespread use of the drugs was discontinued because long-term studies showed that the lower blood sugar level had no impact on longevity or complications from the disease.

5. **Sensitivity.** For a variable to be useful, there must be some reasonable chance that it is related to, or likely to change with, the independent variable under study. As an example, researchers often select a laboratory test result as a measure of effect of a risk factor or therapeutic intervention. For instance, several studies have looked at the effect of formaldehyde on lower respiratory tract disease using measures of pulmonary function as the dependent variable. The choice is reasonable in some respects: pulmonary function can be measured with a high degree of precision and relatively cheaply. The data can be elicited from patients far more easily than by using such alternatives as symptom diaries, which may cause severe problems with compliance. The difficulty is that the effects of formaldehyde may not be detectable with

this measure because they are likely to occur shortly after exposure and dissipate rapidly, and so they have vanished by the time patients arrive at the clinical setting for testing. Also, relatively large changes in pulmonary function, of the order of 20 percent, are required to show any effect on patients' function. For a similar reason, the use of death as an endpoint, however important, is unlikely to be sensitive to any subtle changes resulting from low-level exposure. Of course, if formaldehyde is suspected as a potential human carcinogen, the use of death as a measure, specifically respiratory cancer death, is uniquely appropriate.

The important implication of these considerations is that issues of measurement are central to much research in epidemiology. The choice of an appropriate measure is a complex exercise in compromise. Just as investigators should be aware of the issues involved in this choice, critical readers of the literature should examine closely the variables used in a reported investigation to determine whether they are appropriate for the research goals.

TYPES OF VARIABLES

When considering issues of measurement, it is useful to make a distinction among different types of variables. Although there are various ways to describe the different variables, the important distinction is between those variables that are **categorical**, such as dead/alive, diseased/normal, or Protestant/Catholic/Jewish/other, and those that are **continuous**, like diastolic blood pressure, hemoglobin level, height, and many subjective states, such as pain, disability, or mood. Categorical variables can only take on certain discrete values. By contrast, continuous variables can, in theory, assume an infinite number of values.

Within these broad classes there is often a further subdivision. Categorical variables are classified into *nominal* variables, which are named categories like dead/alive, male/female, or white/Oriental/African, and *ordinal* (ordered) categories like Stage I/Stage II/Stage III cancer or much improved/improved/same/worse/much worse. The distinction between the two is that there is no order implied for nominal variables — whites are no higher or lower than Orientals or Africans. In contrast, there is a clear order implied in ordinal variables (e.g., staging in cancer).

Continuous variables are also divided into two classes. With *interval* variables the distance between points has some quantitative meaning, so that the difference between a blood pressure of 95 mm Hg and 105 mm Hg is the same as the difference between 110 mm Hg and 120 mm Hg. For *ratio* variables, the ratio of two quantities has meaning (e.g., the ratio of two temperatures expressed in degrees Kelvin). These latter two concepts are understood better by considering violations of the rule. A rating scale going from "much below average" to "much above average" is not an interval variable, because the distance between "much below average" and "below average" has no real meaning — it certainly would not be easy to demonstrate, for example, that it is the same as the difference between "average" and "slightly above average." In a similar vein, the ratio of two temperatures expressed in absolute or Kelvin degrees has some meaning, but degrees on the Celsius scale are not ratio variables — 20° C is not twice as hot as 10° C.

The distinction between categorical and continuous variables is important, since it influences nearly every way we think about them, as will become evident in the remainder of this section. However, the difference between nominal and ordinal variables is only important in the application of some slightly esoteric statistical tests that work for ordered categories but not for nominal categories. Similarly, there is virtually no importance to the distinction between interval and ratio variables, so the less said the better.

MEASUREMENT WITH CATEGORICAL VARIABLES

We began this section on measurement with the suggestion that much of the confusion surrounding the carcinogenic risk of many environmental hazards is a result of inadequate attention paid to the quantification of risk. In this section we will develop a number of ways to approach the issue of risk assessment. There are two parts to the question: (1) deciding on the appropriate way to **measure** the health effect, and (2) deciding on some way to express the **association** between the supposed cause and the outcome.

For the moment let us define the issue a little more precisely. Without getting into the specifics of risks from radiation, PCBs, dioxin, ethylene dibromide, Agent Orange, video display terminals, or hydro lines, it would seem apparent that we are being bombarded with all sorts of chemical, electromagnetic, nuclear, and particulate delights that never assaulted our ancestors. That being the case, one possible result of the overall impact of all these insults to the organism would be an increase in the overall rate of cancer over the past century or so. If these pollutants are indeed devastating our health, this should be reflected in a gradual increase in cancer rates as time passes.

As we shall see, this *seems* simple enough, but it isn't. First, should we count all cases of cancer, or all deaths from cancer? After all, to the extent that our therapies are getting better we might actually be curing some folks, which would make the death rate drop even though there may be just as many or even more cases around. On the other hand, we're also getting better at detecting cancer with methods like Pap smears and mammography, which weren't available a few years or decades ago. The effect of this might be to inflate the apparent number of cases in recent years, although it would have less impact on deaths, since by the time someone dies from it, cancer is fairly obvious.

For convenience and convention we call the counting of cases the measurement of **frequency**, and the counting of deaths the measurement of **impact**. We will explore the issue of the overall effect of the environment using both these measures, by examining the risk of cancer in the 1930s and the 1980s to see if we can detect the effect of a (questionably) deteriorating environment.

MEASURES OF FREQUENCY

Measures of frequency focus on the **occurrence** of disease as opposed to the sequelae of disease (in particular, death). There are a number of ways one can approach the counting of disease. The choice is based on the unpleasant reality that it takes some time to do a study, and while the clock is ticking, new folks are unfortunately developing a disease at the same time that some lucky souls are being cured of it (at least for some diseases) and others are dying of it. All this coming-and-going in and out of the study wreaks havoc with any attempt to count who actually has the disease. To overcome this state of affairs, epidemiologists have worked out a few standard ways of counting bodies, warm or otherwise.

To return to our original problem, let's suppose we wish to count all cases of cancer (of all types) in Canada in 1987. Having agreed on the criteria for diagnosis and carefully set up a sampling frame that is perfectly representative of the population of Canada, or, alternatively, having developed a reporting mechanism for all cases in Canada, we now start counting on January 1 and stop on December 31. All the counts come pouring in, and the systems analysts and statisticians are rubbing their hands in glee at all the years of prospective employment ahead. Now the embarrassing questions emerge.

To illustrate the difficulty, let's examine what happened at the cancer reporting center in Plumcoulee, Manitoba. There are a total of 200 people in this farming community, a fact that we'll need to know later. The reports to the center are shown in Table 3-1.

It is obvious from the table that we can get wildly different estimates of the amount of cancer in Plumcoulee depending on how we choose to do the counting. If we just look at the number of cases around at any point in time, we find four in January, three in December, and eight in July. If we count the total number of folks who were reported this year, the answer is 12. If we count the number of new cases in 1987, it's eight. Finally, there were six deaths from cancer in that year.

There are, however, some standard ways to report the data, as we'll discuss in this section.

TABLE 3-1   Reports of Cancer, Plumcoulee, Manitoba

Patient	Jan	Feb	Mar	Apr	May	Jun	Jul	Aug	Sep	Oct	Nov	Dec
1						X						
2			D							X		
3												
4											X	
5						D C						
6		D						X				
7		C										
8					D							
9					D						X	
10											D	
11						D				C		
12	D			X								

D = first diagnosis; ▬▬ = with disease; C = cured; X = died

INCIDENCE

Incidence is defined as follows:

$$\text{Incidence} = \frac{\text{Number of new cases in a fixed time period}}{\text{Number of people at risk}}$$

Usually the period of study is chosen to be 1 year, in which case we speak of the **annual incidence**. In Plumcoulee (see Table 3-1) there were eight new cases of cancer in 1987. If we had decided to focus on the 3-month incidence, there were three new cases from January to March.

The denominator, or number of people at risk, is not quite 200 people because patients 1,3,4, and 7 already had cancer and thus could not be counted as "at risk"; this reduces the denominator to 196. Thus the annual incidence is:

$$\text{Annual Incidence} = \frac{8}{196} = 0.0408 \text{ cases per year}$$

Usually the incidence of disease is much lower than in this example, and the correction for preexisting cases is unnecessary. Further, to make things more readable, incidence is often cited as cases per 1,000 (in this example, 40.8 cases per 1,000 per year), or even as cases per million per year for very rare disorders.

PREVALENCE

If we are planning screening programs, disease incidence is of immediate interest. However, if we are concerned with the provision of services for people with the disease, such as palliative care, our immediate concern is "How many people actually have the disease at any point in time?" This quantity is called the **prevalence**, which is defined as follows:

$$\text{Prevalence} = \frac{\text{Number of people with the disease}}{\text{Number of people at risk}}$$

In contrast to incidence, prevalence is determined at a single point in time. Still considering the data from Table 3-1, perhaps the most rational point in time to choose is the middle of 1987, or July 1. Looking at the table, we find that patients 2, 3, 4, 6, 8, and 9 had cancer at this time. Patient 5 was cured sometime in July, and should be counted on July 1, whereas patient 11 was diagnosed in July and would likely not enter the count. This leaves a total of seven cases in the numerator.

Again the denominator is not quite 200. By July 1, patients 1 and 12 were deceased, so the denominator is only 198. Finally, the prevalence is:

$$\text{Prevalence} = \frac{7}{198} = 0.0354 = 35.4 \text{ per } 1,000$$

PERIOD PREVALENCE

A close analogy to the incidence is the **period prevalence**, which is based on the number of people with the disease over a defined period of time (usually 1 year). The formal definition is:

$$\text{Prevalence} = \frac{\text{Number of people with the disease over the time period}}{\text{Number of people at risk over the time period}}$$

The calculation of annual prevalence in our example from Table 3-1 is straightforward. There are 12 people identified as having cancer in that year, and 200 at risk, so the period prevalence is simply $12/200 = 0.06 = 60$ per 1,000. If we were to calculate the quarterly prevalence for the first quarter of the year, we would include only patients 1, 2, 3, 4, 6, 7, and 12; the period prevalence for 3 months is therefore $7/200 = 0.035 = 35$ per 1,000.

RELATION BETWEEN PREVALENCE AND INCIDENCE

The previous definitions were slightly different in dimensions. Incidence is based on a fixed time period, and is quoted per month or year. However, prevalence is calculated at a single point in time. It happens that the two quantities have an interesting relationship, which involves the average duration of disease:

$$\text{Prevalence} = \text{Incidence} \times \text{Duration}$$

It's not easy to demonstrate the relationship mathematically, but it is easy to show that it is reasonable. Think of a chronic, but relatively nonlethal disease like rheumatoid arthritis (RA). Once an individual acquires the disease, he/she carries it until death, so the duration is calculated by subtracting the average age at onset from the expected life span. Thus, each new case of RA is added to the pool of prevalent cases, and although relatively few cases may be added each year, there are a large number of prevalent cases around. So the prevalence of RA is much greater than annual incidence.

By contrast, the ordinary cold has a duration of a few days at most, and kids can often get more than one per year. In this situation the annual incidence might approach, or even exceed, 1,000 per 1,000. Yet unless there's an epidemic around, relatively few people have a cold at any time, so the prevalence of colds is not nearly as high as the incidence — perhaps 50 per 1,000. Because the duration is very short, the prevalence is much lower than the annual incidence.

The relationship may seem to be of only arcane interest. However, it is often easier to obtain published data on disease prevalence than on incidence; yet if you want to do an intervention or prevention study, it is usually of greater interest to know how many new cases you are likely to get. Through the use of this formula and a reasoned guess at the duration of the disease, you can arrive at a plausible estimate of the number of new cases.

CASE FATALITY RATE

While we're examining the fate of the Plumcoulee patients from Table 3-1, we might as well introduce a term that links disease *frequency*, or the likelihood of developing the disease, to disease *impact*, which is the likelihood of dying from the disease.

First of all we note that a total of six persons from Plumcoulee died of cancer during the study. It is natural to express this quantity in a similar manner to our measures of disease occurrence to form a quantity called the **mortality rate**; which is defined as follows:

$$\text{Mortality Rate} = \frac{\text{Number of deaths from disease in a time period}}{\text{Number of people at risk}}$$

Studying the data from Plumcoulee, we see that six people (patients 1, 2, 4, 6, 9, and 12) died of cancer in 1987. There were 200 people at risk, so the **annual mortality rate** was $6/200 = 0.03$, or 30 per 1,000.

As we shall see in the discussion on measures of impact, this approach is a fairly crude basis for comparison. However, there is another relationship evident from the display. When relating frequency to impact we might wish to study the likelihood that a disease may be fatal. This quantity is called the **case fatality rate**, and is defined as follows:

$$\text{Case Fatality Rate} = \frac{\text{Number of deaths from disease in a time period}}{\text{Number of people with the disease}}$$

In the present example there were 12 people with cancer in Plumcoulee in 1987, and six deaths; the case fatality rate is therefore $6/12 = 50$ percent per year.

MEASURES OF IMPACT

We began this discussion with the idea that one broad way to determine whether all the industrial pollutants have affected human health was to examine the rates of cancer over several decades, to see if any increasing trend was evident. We briefly discussed the advantages and disadvantages of looking at disease frequency (cases of cancer) and disease impact (deaths from cancer).

The impact of disease need not focus entirely on death. For a chronic disease like arthritis, disease impact would more appropriately be calculated using measures of activities of daily living, function, or quality of life. However, for the example we have been pursuing we will focus on mortality. The measurement of mortality has one major advantage over the measurement of frequency, namely that relatively complete archival sources are available and have been for several decades (or for several centuries in Great Britain). Instead of setting up a reporting system such as was proposed for Plumcoulee and allowing it to run for a few decades while we epidemiologists cool our collective heels, we can conduct a retrospective impact study. In this discussion we use actual data, based on Canadian statistics for 1933 and 1973, to examine our research hypothesis that the increased level of chemical, radiologic, and particulate pollution in Canada in the intervening 40 years has led to an increase in the observed rate of death from cancer.

MORTALITY RATE

To test this hypothesis, let's turn to our desk copy of Canadian statistics. We look up the appropriate sections and compile the data (Table 3-2). To make the comparison easier, it makes sense to work out the number of deaths per 1,000 population. This is called the annual mortality rate, which is defined as follows:

$$\text{Annual Mortality Rate} = \frac{\text{Number of deaths in a year}}{\text{Total population}}$$

For 1933 the annual mortality rate is 11,056 per 10,500,000, or 1.05 per 1,000. For 1973 the annual mortality rate is 44,877 per 21,400,000, or 2.10 per 1,000.

From these data it would appear that the rate of cancer has nearly doubled in 40 years. We may conclude that perhaps there is evidence of a significant health effect of pollutants. Nevertheless there are a number of steps we can take to refine the comparison.

PROPORTIONAL MORTALITY RATE

We were in the fortunate position when we calculated the mortality rate to have a good estimate of the denominator, or the population at risk. Federal census takers in the Western world go to great pains and expense to determine how many people there are in the country in given years (perhaps so they can ensure complete tax returns to pay for the census). However, in many situations where research is conducted on subpopulations (e.g., workers exposed to welding fumes or residents near a landfill site) it would be very difficult or impossible to determine on the basis of existing records how many people were in the denominator in a given year.

On the other hand, it is much easier to determine the cause of death of all the people in a population who died, because death certificates are a legal necessity. We can reason that if pollutants are causing more cancer in 1973

TABLE 3-2   Canadian Cancer Statistics

	1933	1973
Total population	10,500,000	21,400,000
Deaths from cancer	11,056	44,877

than they did in 1933, proportionately more deaths should be caused by cancer than by other causes in 1973 than in 1933. This approach is called the **proportional mortality rate** or **PMR**. It requires no knowledge of the people at risk, only mortality data. The PMR is defined as follows:

$$PMR = \frac{\text{Number of deaths from a particular cause}}{\text{Total number of deaths}}$$

It turns out that in 1933 there were a total of 122,850 deaths recorded in Canada. In 1973, 236,200 deaths were recorded. The resultant PMRs are shown in Table 3-3.

It appears that the same trend to higher mortality rates in 1973 is present in these data. Of course one alternative explanation is that proportionately more people were dying of cancer in 1973 simply because fewer people were dying from everything else. This makes some sense because tuberculosis, diphtheria, and other serious infectious diseases were present in 1933 but absent in 1973. Certainly there is some evidence that this may be occurring; males born in 1933 had a life expectancy of 41.1 years, whereas men born in 1973 had a life expectancy of 68.2 years.

This example also nicely illustrates the strengths and weaknesses of the PMR method. Its strength is that it can be applied in situations in which only minimal data are available; its weakness is that a high PMR is always open to two interpretations: (1) more deaths from the cause of interest or (2) fewer deaths from everything else.

AGE-SPECIFIC MORTALITY

In general, cancer is a disease of old age. Although a few young persons die of cancer, in most circumstances there is a period of a few decades between exposure to some cancer-causing agent and the onset of the disease. This must be kept in mind when contrasting 1933 with 1973; not only might more people have died from other causes in 1933, as we mentioned previously, but also more people might have died young from other causes and not lived long enough to develop cancer.

To determine if this reasoning results in an alternative explanation for the higher observed cancer mortality in 1973, we could look only at the death rate from cancer in older people (e.g., older than 75 years of age). We could

TABLE 3–3   **Proportional Mortality Rates for Cancer**

	1933	1973
Total deaths	122,850	236,200
Deaths from cancer	11,056	44,877
Proportional mortality rate	9.0%	19.0%

then calculate the cancer mortality rate in this age segment. The result is called the **age-specific mortality rate**, which is defined as follows:

$$\text{Age-Specific MR} = \frac{\text{Number of deaths in a particular age range}}{\text{Total number of deaths in a particular age range}}$$

Let's work this example through. In 1933 there were 5,126 Canadians older than 75; in this group there were 110 cancer deaths. Therefore the age-specific mortality rate is $110/5,126 = 21.5$ per 1,000. Similar data from 1973 indicate that there were 915 cancer deaths among the 35,295 Canadians over age 75, which results in an age-specific mortality rate of $915/35,295 = 25.9$ per 1,000.

These rates are indeed a little closer than the overall mortality rates we looked at earlier, thereby suggesting that a partial explanation for the differences is simply that people were dying of other causes in 1933 and were not living long enough to develop cancer. However, it is unfortunate that in order to make this comparison it was necessary to ignore most of the data.

STANDARDIZED MORTALITY RATE

The discussion on age-specific mortality rate suggested that if we restricted our view to those individuals who survived long enough to be at risk of developing cancer, there was a smaller difference in cancer rates between 1933 and 1973 than was evident when we simply looked at overall mortality. The difference between the two sets of data reflects (1) the influence of age on mortality rates from a specific disease, and (2) differences in the age distributions between the Canadian population in 1933 and 1973.

Most diseases show a strong relationship with age. Risk from chronic diseases like heart disease and cancer increases with age, whereas infectious diseases are more common in the young. Even pedestrian mortality shows a strong bimodal distribution with age, and strikes the very young, who lack awareness of the dangers of traffic, and the very old, who can no longer see and hear danger as well as before (or run as fast!).

Because of the strong influence of age on disease mortality rates, any comparison between two different populations is considerably strengthened by correcting for the differences in age distribution. This approach is called the **standardized mortality rate** or **SMR**, and builds on the age-specific mortality rate. Having broken down the deaths in the population of interest by age and created age-specific mortality rates, we then use them with the distribution of age in a reference or standard population to create an overall projected mortality rate. There are four basic steps in the process:

1. Calculate the age-specific mortality rate for each age range in the population of interest.

2. Multiply this rate by the number of people in the age range in the standard population. This then determines the number of individuals in the standard population who would die from the disease.
3. Add up the total number of projected deaths across all age levels of the standard population.
4. Finally, convert this to a mortality rate by dividing by the total numbers in the standard population.

For example, to compare the cancer mortality in 1933 and 1973, we will project them both onto a reference population distribution (in this case the population distribution of Canada in 1970, but any year could have been chosen). The method is illustrated in Table 3-4.

After this lengthy process we then can determine that the standardized mortality rate for cancer deaths for 1933 is 2,510 per 1 million, or 2.51 per 1,000. Similar calculations can be performed for cancer deaths in 1973 and from all other causes in both 1933 and 1973, always using the 1970 population as the standard. These calculations are shown in Table 3-5.

TABLE 3-4   Calculations for Standardized Mortality Rate

1 Age Range	2 1933 Pop.	3 Cancer Deaths	4 Age-Specific Mortality (Col. 3 ÷ Col. 2)	5 1970 Pop.	6 Standard Deaths (Col. 4 × Col. 5)
0–4	49,113	2	0.000041	84,416	3.44
5–9	42,014	4	0.000095	98,204	9.35
.					
.					
.					
75–79	2,891	41	0.014182	18,871	267.6
80–84	1,403	40	0.028510	11,241	320.5
>84	832	29	0.034856	7,435	259.2
Total				1,000,000	2,510

TABLE 3-5   Standardized Mortality Rates per 1,000

	1933	1973
Cancer	2.51	3.10
All other causes	15.12	8.91

Some of our suspicions are therefore correct. People indeed died at a much faster rate from other causes in 1933 than in 1973 — 15.12 per 1,000 versus 8.91 per 1,000, respectively. There nevertheless appears to be an excess cancer risk persisting in 1973 of about 20 percent (3.10 versus 2.51 per 1,000). However, this is considerably less than the doubled risk originally calculated using the unstandardized mortality rates.

SUMMARY

The standardized mortality rate is about the best estimate of the mortality arising from a particular cause, and is virtually a prerequisite for any comparison across different populations. Proportional mortality rates are a weak alternative, useful only in situations in which there are no denominator data available.

It should be kept in mind that the application of SMRs corrects for the confounding effect of age, and possibly of sex differences, but that's all. To conclude that *any* observed difference results from a particular cause requires the elimination of all other possible causes. The point is nicely illustrated by a final run at the 1933-1973 comparison.

The difficulty arises from the use of a historical control, as described in *Research Methodology*. To conclude that the observed difference between 1933 and 1973 is caused by industrial pollution requires that we eliminate from suspicion all the other differences between 1933 and 1973. One difference in particular is staring us in the face—cigarette smoking. Smoking per capita has increased steadily from the turn of the century until recent times, and cigarettes are a known and strong causal factor in lung cancer. These facts suggest that we may further understand the cause of the increase of cancer deaths from 1933 to 1973 by separating respiratory cancer from cancers of all other sites (since the latter are only weakly related to smoking). If we do this, and calculate SMRs for respiratory cancer and other sites, all the differences between 1973 and 1933 can be accounted for by a sevenfold difference in respiratory cancer rates (Table 3-6). This of course doesn't prove that smoking, rather than pollution, is the cause of the increase. However, it does suggest that there is no general impact of air, water, and foodborne chemicals on human health reflected in cancer rates.

TABLE 3-6   Respiratory Cancers vs Cancers from All Other Sites*

	1933	1973
Respiratory	0.09	0.69
Other sites	2.42	2.41
Total	2.51	3.20

* Standardized mortality rates per 1,000

MEASURES OF ASSOCIATION WITH CATEGORICAL VARIABLES

We began this discussion with the assertion that much of our fear about cancer and the environment was a result of inadequate quantification of the additional risk. To this point we have dwelt on measurement issues and sought means to measure the health effects in an unbiased manner. We now wish to explore methods to measure the *strength of association* between two variables.

We have already used some rough-and-ready measures of association. We found in the last section that there was a sevenfold higher risk of respiratory cancer in 1973 than in 1933. We could restate the data in two other ways: (1) the risk of respiratory cancer increased from 0.09 per 1,000 to 0.69 per 1,000, or (2) there was a risk of cancer of 0.60 per 1,000 attributed to the different circumstances in 1973 and 1933. In the next few examples we will formalize these concepts.

Let's begin with a new example that is related to therapeutic benefit. The issue is the relationship between cholesterol and heart disease. For a long time a strong association between serum cholesterol and heart disease has been known; however, the implications of this finding were not clear. Did a high level of cholesterol "cause" heart disease, or was it simply a marker of a certain genetic predisposition? The key issue has been whether it could be demonstrated that lowering cholesterol levels by diet or drugs would reduce the rate of heart disease.

This was finally demonstrated in 1985 by the Coronary Primary Prevention Trial (CPPT), a randomized trial that was conducted at a number of clinics in North America. The researchers began by screening nearly half a million men to find a group of 3,900 who had very high serum cholesterol levels (above 256 mg per deciliter) but as yet no evidence of disease. The men also had to comply with a fierce regimen. The drug, called cholestyramine, was foul-smelling, foul-tasting, and gut-wrenching, and had to be taken in water six times per day. The researchers eventually found their bunch of docile souls who would go along with the treatment. They were randomized into two groups (the placebo was concocted to taste just as bad) and followed for 7 to 10 years. After the dust settled there were 30 cardiac deaths in the drug group and 38 in the control group, figures that were statistically significant. There was no overall difference in death rates, but this won't concern us. The ways in which these data might be displayed are discussed next.

RELATIVE RISK

The data from the cholestyramine study appear in Table 3-7. The **relative risk**, as the name implies, is a measure of the likelihood of occurrence of the target event (death or disease) in those exposed and not exposed to the agent of interest. It is defined as follows:

$$\text{Relative Risk} = \frac{\text{Mortality rate (or incidence) in exposed group}}{\text{Mortality rate (or incidence) in unexposed group}}$$

TABLE 3–7   Data from Cholestyramine Study

	Cardiac Deaths	Alive	Total
Cholestyramine	30	1,870	1,900
Placebo	38	1,868	1,906

Mortality rates in the two groups are 30 per 1,900 and 38 per 1,906. Therefore, the relative risk from cholestyramine is $30/1,900 \div 38/1,906 = 0.792$. To put it another way, the risk of cardiac death in the treated group was $1.00 - 0.792$, or 21 percent lower than in the placebo group, a risk reduction of 21 percent.

The data can be presented in another way. We could turn the question around and ask what the relative risk of cardiac death resulting from the absence of a drug is. This relative risk is the inverse of the previous calculation: $38/1,906 \div 30/1,900 = 1.26$.

ETIOLOGIC FRACTION

Closely related to the notion of risk reduction is a concept called the **etiologic fraction (EF)**. When considering a risk factor for a disease, in this case high cholesterol levels, we are interested in what fraction of the cases of cardiac death has high cholesterol levels as its etiology. Since there were 38 deaths in this cohort when high cholesterol levels were present, and 30 deaths when this risk factor was absent, we could define the proportion of cardiac deaths, or the EF, as follows:

$$EF = \frac{\text{Mortality in exposed group} - \text{Mortality in unexposed group}}{\text{Mortality in exposed group}}$$

For the CPPT trial (see Table 3-7) the etiologic fraction is $(38 - 30) \div 38 = 21$ percent. This is the same number as, although a different concept than, the risk reduction we calculated earlier.

ATTRIBUTABLE RISK

The relative risk gives some indication of the increased risk (in the case of a risk factor) or benefit (in the case of a therapy) in relative terms. However, we would often like to examine the actual increase or reduction in incidence or mortality attributed to the cause. This is called the **attributable risk (AR)**, and is defined as follows:

AR = Mortality rate (or incidence) in exposed group − Mortality rate (or incidence) in unexposed group

In the cholestyramine example (see Table 3-7) the attributable risk of cardiac death (attributable to the absence of the benefit derived from cholestyramine) is $38/1,906 - 30/1,900 = 4.1$ per 1,000.

The example nicely illustrates the important differences between the two concepts of relative risk and attributable risk. The CPPT trial began with a highly selected cohort of people with very high cholesterol levels, followed them for a long time (7 to 10 years), and indeed demonstrated a statistically significant risk reduction of 21 percent. However, this amounted to a reduction in risk of cardiac death of only four per 1,000, compared with a total rate of death in both groups of about 70 per 1,000.

RELATIVE ODDS

The concepts of association we have discussed so far work well for most situations in which we wish to examine the effect of a particular risk factor on the subsequent occurrence of disease. However, there is one study design, the case-control study (see *Research Methodology*), in which things don't quite fit. Case-control studies are used in situations in which the likelihood of developing disease is low, or there is a long latency before the onset of disease. Typically, both these conditions apply to the investigation of risk factors in cancer. In these circumstances we assemble a group of people with the disease (cases) and an appropriate set of people without disease (controls), usually of the same size, and we examine the exposure of the two groups to the risk factor of interest.

As one example, continuing our cancer theme, Table 3-8 was derived from one of the original studies linking lung cancer to smoking.

The fact that the rate of lung cancer overall is so high is a sure clue that we are dealing with a case-control study, since if these data were based on a cohort study that assembled persons who did and didn't smoke, we would arrive at the alarming conclusion that the overall rate of lung cancer was about 34 percent. However, if we continue along the lines we had done previously, we could calculate a risk of cancer in the exposed group of $659/684$, or 96 percent, and in the unexposed group of $984/1,332$, or 74 percent. The relative risk of lung cancer is then, using the previous methods, $0.96 \div 0.74 = 1.30$. Although the final result seems plausible, the intermediate steps are insane because of the nature of the design. In fact,

TABLE 3-8   Lung Cancer and Smoking

	Cases	Controls	Total
Smoker	659 (A)	984 (B)	1,643
Nonsmoker	25 (C)	348 (D)	373
Total	684	1,332	2,016

lung cancer is much rarer than we have made it out to be; the controls without cancer are sampled from a much larger population of healthy folks than are the cases.

Although we cannot calculate from these data an actual risk of getting lung cancer, we can frame things in a different way. We begin with the cases and play a gambling game, asking the odds that this person was exposed to the suspected carcinogen. When a gambler says that the odds of a candidate's being elected are 1:4, he is saying that the probability of his being elected is one-quarter that of his not being elected, and since these probabilities add to one, a little mental arithmetic shows that the probability that this candidate will be elected is 20 percent. Similarly, the odds that an individual with lung cancer was exposed to tobacco are $A/C = 659/25 = 26.4$; and the odds that an individual in the control group was exposed is $B/D = 984/348 = 2.83$. The **relative odds** of lung cancer from tobacco exposure are then:

$$\text{Relative Odds} = \frac{\text{Odds of exposure for cases}}{\text{Odds of exposure for controls}} = \frac{A/C}{B/D}$$
$$= 26.4/2.83$$
$$= 9.33$$

DIAGNOSTIC TESTS

The twentieth century has seen dramatic changes in disease patterns in the Western world. Since the advent of effective antibiotics, vaccines, and, perhaps most important, adequate nutrition and sanitation, most people in industrialized countries can look forward to a full life. Our present preoccupation is with chronic, lifestyle-related diseases for which there are unlikely to be any "magic bullets" in the foreseeable future.

One result of these changes is that epidemiologists have moved away from their historical roots in the study of epidemics to such diverse activities as the study of occupational risks or trials of therapeutic agents, in order to maintain employment. (One result of this shift in employment patterns is that books such as this are now required to tell health professionals what epidemiologists do.)

However, thanks to a new infectious disease, AIDS, that has all the devastating characteristics of the traditional scourges of mankind like cholera and the black plague, epidemiologists find themselves the center of attention at cocktail parties. We need not devote any space in this section to describing the natural history, prevalence, modes of transmission, or risk factors of AIDS — these are taught to elementary school students. However, we will use this disease as an instructive example of a measurement problem, the application of diagnostic tests.

There are now two high-risk populations for AIDS — homosexuals because of sexual contact and street drug users because of the sharing of contaminated needles. Before the advent of adequate screening tests, there was a third high-risk segment — people requiring blood transfusions for any reason. In particular, a significant number of hemophiliacs acquired AIDS as a result of their exposure to large numbers of transfusions. However, since 1985 all blood products are routinely screened for AIDS using the enzyme linked immunosorbent assay (ELISA) test.

As diagnostic tests go, ELISA is a very good one indeed. This is fortunate, because the consequences of the test are severe. If an individual has AIDS antibodies, there is at least a 30 percent chance of developing the disease, and AIDS has nearly a 100 percent mortality. The consequences of a false positive are also severe. If we tell someone he/she has antibodies when this isn't the case, we are causing massive anxiety and lifestyle changes. Conversely, if we miss blood products containing antibodies, the chance of infecting someone is high.

Let us examine the performance of this test in two populations: (1) in a homosexual population, in which the prevalence of AIDS antibodies is about 50 percent, and (2) in routine screening of blood donations, in which the prevalence of antibodies is about 0.2 percent.

TRUE POSITIVE, FALSE POSITIVE, TRUE NEGATIVE, AND FALSE NEGATIVE RATES

Let us imagine that the ELISA test is being used as a diagnostic test for a high-risk population, e.g., homosexuals in New York City. Actual figures for this group indicate that the prevalence of the AIDS antibody is about 50 percent.

To examine the test performance, we could screen a group of individuals and compare the test result with their true status. Truth isn't easy to come by, but in this case there is a more expensive, but virtually perfect test called the Western blot test. We could take samples from the group and perform both tests on the samples. If we were to screen 1,000 individuals with the test and compare the test result to the "gold standard," the results would be similar to those found in Table 3-9.

TABLE 3-9   Results of ELISA vs Western Blot Test in Screening of 1,000 Homosexuals from New York City

	Gold Standard (Western Blot)		
	Antibodies	No Antibodies	Total
ELISA Positive	498 (A)	4 (B)	502
Negative	10 (C)	488 (D)	498
Total	508	492	1,000

The characteristics of tests are usually described in terms of the letters (A, B, C, D) in the four cells of the table. One way of describing the test's performance is as follows:

True Positive Rate $= \dfrac{\text{People with positive test and disease}}{\text{All people with disease}}$

$$= A/(A + C) = 498/508$$
$$= 98.03 \text{ percent}$$

False Negative Rate $= \dfrac{\text{People with negative test and disease}}{\text{All people with disease}}$

$$= C/(A + C) = 10/508$$
$$= 1.97 \text{ percent}$$

True Negative Rate $= \dfrac{\text{People with negative test and no disease}}{\text{All people without disease}}$

$$= D/(B + D) = 488/492$$
$$= 99.19 \text{ percent}$$

False Positive Rate $= \dfrac{\text{People with positive test and no disease}}{\text{All people without disease}}$

$$= B/(B + D) = 4/492$$
$$= 0.81 \text{ percent}$$

SENSITIVITY AND SPECIFICITY

Another way of describing the test's characteristics has its origins in the biochemistry laboratory. We speak of **sensitivity** — how sensitive the test is at detecting disease — and **specificity** — how good the test is at rejecting samples that are not diseased. Let's use the data from Table 3-9.

The test sensitivity is a measure of the test's ability to detect people with the disease, and is measured as follows:

$$\text{Sensitivity} = \frac{\text{Number with disease who have a positive test}}{\text{Number with disease}}$$

$$= A/(A + C) = 498/508$$
$$= 98.03 \ \text{percent}$$

Conversely, the test specificity measures the ability of the test to correctly identify people who do not have the disease, and is measured as follows:

$$\text{Specificity} = \frac{\text{Number without disease who have a negative test}}{\text{Number with disease}}$$

$$= D/(B + D) = 488/492$$
$$= 99.19 \ \text{percent}$$

As you can see, sensitivity is the same as true positive rate, and specificity is the same as true negative rate.

POSITIVE AND NEGATIVE PREDICTIVE VALUE

The descriptions thus far give some picture of the characteristics of the test. However, the denominator for both sensitivity and specificity assumes some knowledge of the true state of affairs, since it is based on people who do or don't have the disease. Clinicians rarely have the luxury of a "gold standard"; if they did, they wouldn't be doing the test. Putting it another way, assume you are about to advise someone who has just received a positive ELISA. Do you tell the individual that he/she has AIDS antibodies? What is the chance that someone with a positive ELISA does not have antibodies? These probabilities are embodied in the concepts of **positive predictive value** and **negative predictive value**, in which the denominators are based on people with positive and negative tests. Again using the data from Table 3-9, these values are measured as follows:

$$\text{Positive Predictive Value} = \frac{\text{People with positive test and disease}}{\text{All people with positive test}}$$

$$= A/(A + B)$$
$$= 498/502$$
$$= 99.20 \text{ percent}$$

$$\text{Negative Predictive Value} = \frac{\text{People with negative test and no disease}}{\text{All people with negative test}}$$

$$= D/(C + D)$$
$$= 488/498$$
$$= 97.99 \text{ percent}$$

RELATIONSHIP BETWEEN PREVALENCE AND PREDICTIVE VALUE

The data we have presented so far give a fairly encouraging picture of the ELISA test. If someone has a positive test, we can be 99.2 percent certain that person really has AIDS antibodies. However, the calculations were based on a situation where the prevalence of antibodies was high (about 50 percent). In different circumstances the picture may not be as rosy. For example, experience in screening blood donations has shown that the prevalence of AIDS antibodies is actually closer to 0.2 percent. As pointed out over 3 decades ago, this change in prevalence may drastically affect the usefulness of the test.

Working out a new contingency table (as in Table 3-9) we now have a prevalence of 0.2 percent; two people out of the 1,000 will have antibodies, and 998 will not. Because the prevalence is so low, imagine screening 1,000,000 units of blood, of which about 2,000 will have antibodies (whether we use 1,000 samples or 1,000,000 does not affect the results at all, it just eliminates decimal points during the calculations). Since the test has a sensitivity of 98.0 percent, $0.98 \times 2,000 = 1,960$ persons will test positive with ELISA (cell A) and 40 will test negative (cell C). Now there will be $1,000,000 - 2,000$, or 998,000 normal units of blood. We know from our previous data that the specificity of the test is 99.2 percent; there will be a total of $0.992 \times 998,000 = 990,016$ normal units that test negative (cell D). Conversely, there will be $998,000 - 990,016 = 7,984$ normal units of blood that have positive ELISA tests (cell C). The new data appear in Table 3-10.

TABLE 3-10   Prevalence of AIDS per 1,000,000 Units of Blood

| | Gold Standard (Western Blot) | | |
	Antibodies	No Antibodies	Total
Positive	1,960 (A)	7,984 (B)	9,944
Negative	40 (C)	990,016 (D)	990,056
Total	2,000	998,000	1,000,000

ELISA (row label for Positive/Negative)

If we now recalculate the predictive values, they look like this:

$$\text{Positive Predictive Value} = 1,960/9,944$$
$$= 19.7 \text{ percent}$$
$$\text{Negative Predictive Value} = 990,016/990,056$$
$$= 99.99 \text{ percent}$$

The picture is now very different than in the first situation. If a person has a negative test, there is virtual certainty that he/she truly is AIDS-negative. However, a positive test is nearly uninterpretable because more than 80 percent of the positive test results come from people who don't have antibodies!

In actual practice any blood that tests positive is sent for a repeat ELISA and a Western blot test. If ELISA remains positive and the Western blot is negative, the blood is discarded but the donor is not told. If they are both positive, the donor is informed and contacts traced.

Thus in general, the prevalence of disease has a profound effect on the usefulness of a test. If the prevalence is low, the positive predictive value of the test is low and the negative predictive value high. Conversely, if the prevalence of disease is very high, the negative predictive value is low but the positive predictive value is high.

BAYES' THEOREM

In the previous discussion we calculated the probability that a person with a positive ELISA had AIDS antibodies, given known data about the prevalence of antibodies and the characteristics of the test. However, we had to take a roundabout route by calculating a new contingency table (see Table 3-10) and then working out the appropriate values. There is an algebraic shortcut, called **Bayes' theorem**, that permits this calculation directly. To do the calculation, we will also introduce some new symbols that frequently appear in the epidemiologic literature:

$$P(D) = \text{Probability of disease before the test}$$
$$= \text{Prevalence} = 0.2 \text{ percent}$$

$$P(T+ \mid D) = \text{Probability of positive test given the disease}$$
$$= \text{Sensitivity} = 98.0 \text{ percent}$$

$$P(T+ \mid \overline{D}) = \text{Probability of positive test given no disease}$$
$$= (1 - \text{Specificity}) = 0.8 \text{ percent}$$

$$P(T- \mid D) = \text{Probability of negative test given the disease}$$
$$= (1 - \text{Sensitivity}) = 2.0 \text{ percent}$$

$$P(T- \mid \overline{D}) = \text{Probability of negative test given no disease}$$
$$= \text{Specificity} = 99.2 \text{ percent}$$

According to Bayes' theorem, the probability of disease given a positive test, $P(D \mid T+)$ (i.e., the positive predictive value), is as follows:

$$P(D \mid T+) = \frac{P(D) \times P(T+ \mid D)}{P(D) \times P(T+ \mid D) + [1.0 - P(D)] \times P(T+ \mid \overline{D})}$$

$$= \frac{0.2 \times 98}{(0.2 \times 98) + (0.8 \times 99.8)} = \frac{19.6}{99.44} = 19.7 \text{ percent}$$

A similar calculation could be done to get the negative predictive value.

Bayes' theorem can also be used in an iterative fashion. If we had a situation involving a series of laboratory tests, we could now calculate the posttest probability for the second, third, and subsequent tests. In each case we would use the calculated posttest probability from the previous test as the pretest probability for the calculation of the next test.

RECEIVER OPERATING CHARACTERISTIC CURVES

One measure that is frequently employed for evaluating the effectiveness of diagnostic systems is the **receiver operating characteristic (ROC)** curve. Particularly popular in radiology, it has roots in electrical engineering and psychophysics.

Imagine a laboratory test that has continuous values, such as cardiac enzymes, and consider the problem of attempting to find an appropriate cut-point where any value above the point is considered a positive (i.e., indicative of myocardial infarction), and any point below is considered negative or normal. If we set the point too high, we will miss a number of mild myocardial infarctions, but will avoid false positives. Conversely, a point set too low will catch all the myocardial infarctions at the cost of filling cardiac care unit beds with normal (non-myocardial infarction) patients. This situation is illustrated in Figure 3-1.

As we move the cut-point from right to left, we will initially pick up true positives and few false positives. However, as we pass the center of the myocardial infarction distribution, the rate of pickup of the false positives will increase, and the true positives decrease, to the point that nearly all the increase is false positives. Plotting the true positive rate on the Y-axis and the false positive rate on the X-axis, we generate the ROC curve, as in Figure 3-2.

The ROC curve has some interesting features. First, we note that a perfect test would pick up only true positives at first, then after the true positive rate is 100 percent, only false positives; this describes a curve going vertically along the Y-axis and then horizontally along the top. Conversely, a useless test picks up both true and false positives at the same rate, and traces out a line at 45 degrees. The extent to which the ROC curve "crowds the corner" is a measure of the value of the test. This is measured by the area between the curve and the 45 degree line. Second, the best cutoff to minimize overall errors occurs when the tangent to the line is at 45 degrees; displaying the data this way therefore permits a rational selection of cutoff. The advantage of the ROC approach is that it permits a clear separation between the intrinsic value of the test, as captured in the area under the curve, and the errors associated with an inappropriate choice of cutoff.

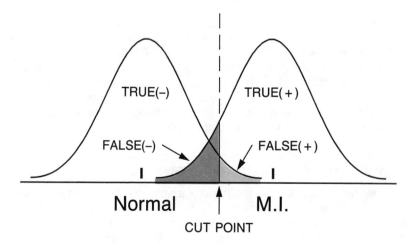

Figure 3-1 Determining the cut-point of a test for myocardial infarction.

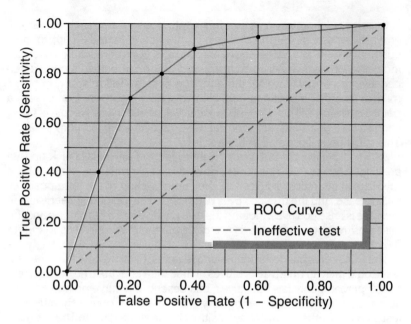

Figure 3-2 ROC curve.

ACCURACY

As yet we have not considered any measure of the overall accuracy of the test. One approach that is very straightforward is to simply sum up the numbers on the diagonal of the table, cells A and D, and place them over the total of all cells. Let's use the data from our two AIDS examples (Tables 3-9 and 3-10).

The overall accuracy of the test, based on data from Table 3-9, is (498 + 488)/1,000 = 98.6 percent. For the lower prevalence situation in Table 3-10, the accuracy is (1,960 + 990,016)/1,000,000 = 99.198 percent. Even though the test is much less useful in the low prevalence case, the accuracy has improved, since the huge numbers of true negatives have predominated in the calculation of accuracy. Because of the possibility of misleading results from this approach, most assessments of accuracy are performed by correcting for chance agreement using a statistic called Cohen's Kappa.

CHANCE CORRECTION USING COHEN'S KAPPA

As we have just seen, the likelihood of agreement between a test result and a "gold standard" is affected by the prevalence of disease. In the extreme case we could consider the application of a clinical sign, right-handedness, to a classical "disease" of Victorian times — self-pollution, or masturbation. Right-handed people are in the majority with about 90 per-

TABLE 3-11 **Prediction of Depression from Test Results**

cent of the population. If we are in a population where everyone does "it," the test will be right 90 percent of the time, without conveying any information whatsoever.

To avoid this trap it is desirable to correct for chance agreement. Taking a little less extreme example, consider the data in Table 3-11, which predict depression as diagnosed by expert interview using DSM-III criteria, from a self-completed questionnaire.

The accuracy, as determined before, is $(A+D)/N = (18+63)/100 = 81$ percent. What agreement would we expect by chance? Chance means that there is, in fact, no association between the two variables. Consider first the A cell. We know that on the average 30 percent of all people in the sample have depression, or 30 people. If there is no association between the two variables, we would expect that the same proportion of people with and without depression would have a positive test, simply equal to the overall proportion of positive tests, or 25 percent. So by chance, 25 percent of the 30 depressed people, or 7.5 people, would be in cell A. Similarly, there should be 75 percent of the nondepressed people, or 52.5 people, in cell D. The agreement expected by chance is $(7.5 + 52.5)/100 = 60$ percent. We actually observed 81 percent. It's not necessary to figure out the numbers in cells B and C because we don't use them in the calculation. The chance corrected agreement, called **Kappa**, is defined as:

$$\text{Kappa} = \frac{\text{Observed agreement} - \text{Agreement by chance}}{1.0 - \text{Agreement by chance}} = \frac{0.81 - 0.60}{1.0 - 0.60}$$

$$= 0.21/0.40 = 0.525$$

As a result, the agreement corrected for chance has been reduced from 81 percent to 53 percent.

MEASUREMENT WITH CONTINUOUS VARIABLES

Historically, epidemiology was concerned with the distribution in time and place of disease epidemics; in more recent times clinical epidemiology has focused on the testing of therapies directed to prolonging life by reducing the incidence of such catastrophic events as heart attacks and strokes. In these situations the unit of analysis is the case of disease or death, and measurement issues focus on the verification of presence or absence of disease.

However, physicians and epidemiologists are increasingly coming to recognize that, for many diseases, there is little to be gained in *quantity* of life from foreseeable advances in biomedicine and there is much more potential for gain in *quality* of life. Innovations such as palliative care and geriatric medicine are explicitly not directed to the cure of disease or extension of life; rather, they are an attempt to improve the quality of life.

From the perspective of epidemiology, research in this area presents new measurement challenges. The measurement of quality of life is a new science; different methods proliferate, and seldom yield the same results. There is possibly more error of measurement than might be expected in categorical measures like diagnosis. Conventional approaches to evaluation of measures, such as comparison with a "gold standard," are inapplicable, because no such criterion currently exists, and no clinical equivalent of the autopsy or biopsy will ever be available. Epidemiologists must acquire new skills, borrowed from such disciplines as psychology, education, and economics, in order to understand and contribute to the development of these measures.

With rare exceptions, these outcomes are based on continuous measurement, originating in rating scales or checklists completed by observers or patients. Approaches to the measurement of association with these measures involve unfamiliar concepts like reliability and construct validity. Usually analysis is conducted using parametric statistics, which assume an interval level of measurement, and normal (bell-shaped) distributions. This section briefly reviews some of these concepts. We are not trying to be comprehensive; instead, we will recommend additional readings for readers who wish to venture further.

MEASURES OF ASSOCIATION

To examine the issues of measurement with continuous variables, we will use an example from rheumatology. The issues here are prototypical of the issues we raised in the beginning of this discussion. The diseases of rheumatology — rheumatic arthritis, osteoarthritis, ankylosing spondylitis, and lupus — are rarely fatal, but often are severely incapacitating because they inflict pain, deformity, and dysfunction on their victims. To examine the efficacy of their therapies, rheumatologists have developed a large number of measures of disease severity. Some emerge from the laboratory, such as erythrocyte sedimentation rate and rheumatoid factor, but appear to have little relationship with clinical measures of function. Some appear to be "objective" clinical descriptions of disease process, such as counts of involved joints or erosion counts (from observations of bone erosions on hand roentgenograms) and walk times. On closer scrutiny, however, these objective descriptions appear to have a great deal of variation among observers and relatively little relationship with measures of the patient's function. Finally, some measures are based on the patients' own assessment of their function and health, and run the gamut from a simple 10 cm line (called a visual analog scale, presumably to obscure its simplicity) on which the patient puts a mark to indicate his perceived health, to indices of function containing tens or hundreds of questions.

To make sense of this potpourri, it is essential to review empirical evidence that the measures are doing what was intended by their makers. When these questions are examined, the evidence falls into two broad classes. The researcher assessing **reliability** asks whether the measures are giving the same answer over different situations (e.g., different observers or the same observer on two occasions separated by a short time interval). The researcher studying **validity** asks whether the measure is assessing what is intended. Does the index of function related by the patient really assess function, or is the score related to the patient's mood, social status, or whatever?

Because the measures are continuous, we cannot simply place the data into a 2 × 2 table as we used before. (We could do this, but the shoehorn act comes at an awful cost of loss of information, e.g., any height above 5'6" [168 cm] is classified as tall.) Instead we must measure the degree to which an individual who is high on one measure or occasion is high on a second measure or occasion, and the converse. The methods to develop these measures are explored further in the next discussions.

PEARSON CORRELATION

By far the most common measure of association for continuous variables is the **Pearson product-moment correlation**. It was invented in the early 1900s by one of the founders of modern statistics. The correlation is based on the idea of fitting the data by a straight line, as illustrated in Figure 3-3.

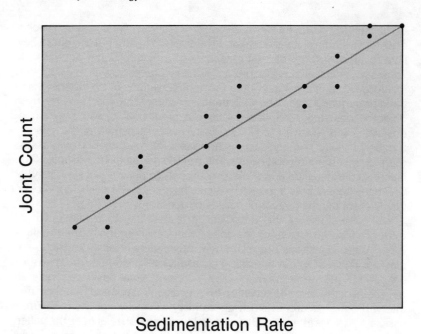

Figure 3-3 Association between erythrocyte sedimentation rate and a measure of active joints in patients with rheumatoid arthritis.

The Pearson correlation is a number between −1 and +1. It equals 0 if there is no relationship, and 1 if there is a perfect linear (straight line) relationship. There is one minor addition: if the slope is negative, that is, if the joint count decreases with increasing sedimentation rate, the correlation is preceded by a minus sign. Therefore a perfect negative relationship has a correlation of −1. Pearson correlations of various sizes are pictured in Figure 3-4.

As you can see, the more the individual points deviate from the straight line, the lower the correlation. With a perfect correlation (+1 or −1), all the points fall on the line. It should be evident from Figure 3-4 that a correlation of 0.8 indicates a fairly good association. Conversely, a correlation of anything less than 0.3 is hardly worth the excitement, statistically significant or not.

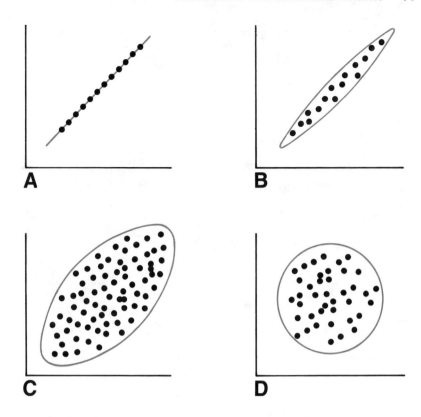

Figure 3-4 Correlations of various sizes. *A*, r = 1; *B*, r = 0.9; *C*, r = 0.5; *D*, r = 0.

INTRACLASS CORRELATION

The Pearson correlation is a perfectly appropriate measure of association to express the degree of linear relationship between two variables. However, under certain circumstances we demand a more stringent measure of association. This situation usually arises in the measurement of agreement between observers, when we don't simply want assurance that a patient scoring high by one observer will also be scored high by the other observer; we want to be sure that the observers are actually giving similar numbers.

Suppose we recruited two rheumatologists to examine hand joints on a series of patients with rheumatoid arthritis and work out the total number of inflamed or swollen joints (Fig. 3-5). It could happen that one observer set very much lower thresholds for what he chose to call "inflamed" than the other, so that for every patient his total was exactly two more (i.e., if one observer said 12 joints, the second said 10, and if one said four, the other said two).

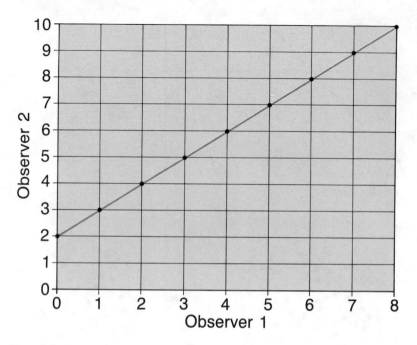

Figure 3-5 The number of hand joints judged as inflamed by two rheumatologists for various patients.

The Pearson correlation simply demands that there is a strong association between the raters — the highest scoring patients for Observer 1 are also the highest for Observer 2, and the lowest for Observer 1 are the lowest for Observer 2. Since this is the case and the points all lie exactly on a straight line, we would get a Pearson correlation of +1. However, by most standards the agreement is terrible; the observers never give the patient the same count.

To get around this problem, the Pearson correlation has been replaced in most circles by the **intraclass correlation (ICC)**. The intraclass correlation is still expressed as a number between 0 and 1; however, the ICC measures not only the *association* between the raters, but also the *agreement.*

Although much is made of the difference between association and agreement and the relative advantages of the intraclass correlation over the Pearson correlation, in most real-world situations the major variability in the data is from apparently random error. Under these circumstances the two measures give identical results. Furthermore, if we treat a 2×2 table as a series of points having values of $(1,1)$, $(0,0)$, $(1,0)$, or $(0,1)$, the intraclass correlation and Kappa yield identical results. For once we can get convergence among differing approaches.

RELIABILITY

Reliability is, as we indicated, a measure of the extent to which a measure is reproducible, or gives the same results, over different situations (e.g., different observers or different days). However, this reproducibility is defined in a very special way by comparing the variability across situations (error variance) to the true variability among patients (patient variance). The reliability coefficient is defined as follows:

$$\text{Reliability} = \frac{\text{Variance due to patients}}{\text{Variance due to patients} + \text{Error variance}}$$

In other words, the reliability expresses the proportion of the variability in the measures that is caused by true variability among patients. The implication of this definition is that if the patients we are studying are truly homogeneous with respect to the attribute of interest, the reliability of the measure will be near 0; conversely, if there is great variability among patients, there will likely be higher reliability. The reliability is a measure of the extent to which we can *differentiate* among patients on a particular attribute.

Although this definition is a bit hard for egalitarian folks to accept, it rests on the simple premise that the goal of measurement is to distinguish among people on a particular attribute. If all the people in the population have the same value of a particular quantity, why bother to measure it? Simply assume that the next person will have that value too.

It is not too difficult to demonstrate that the phenomenon is completely analogous to the discussion about the effect of prevalence on the performance of a diagnostic test. Reliability is like the chance corrected accuracy of a test. If the prevalence of disease drops, this is analogous to the patient population becoming more similar, and the reliability of the continuous measure and the accuracy of the test both fall.

There are some other terms usually associated with reliability, most of which are self-explanatory. **Interobserver** reliability examines the degree of agreement among different observers. **Test-retest** reliability involves administering a test or measure to a group of patients on two different occasions and examining the correlation. **Split-halves** reliability is used in longer tests, and involves splitting the test items into two halves at random and examining the correlations between subscores from the two halves of the test.

There are a number of other specific forms of reliability, but this should give you the idea.

VALIDITY

FACE AND CONTENT VALIDITY

Having demonstrated that a measure is reproducible, it remains to be shown that it is measuring what is intended. Sometimes this is straightforward and noncontroversial; for example, to show that a mercury manometer is measuring blood pressure validly, one might compare blood pressure values obtained this way with direct measures of arterial blood pressure.

More frequently the situation is not so straightforward. How do you demonstrate that your new measure is really assessing self-concept, illness behavior, locus of control, or quality of life? One way is to argue that it measures trait X because trait X is what it measures, an argument that is invoked in a variety of forms for the measurement of intelligence. However, this approach is a little circular; a variation on the theme that is a little less egocentric is to approach a group of experts and ask them whether the measure looks like a reasonable measure of the concept as they understand it. This approach is termed **face validity**. You could also ask them if the measure appears to contain all the important concepts, behaviors, and elements of the concept. If the answer is "yes," you have also attained content validity.

There are better approaches to the measurement of content validity. For example, you might observe patients to see behaviors, interview them or review records, or base the instrument on previous reported measures. All of these strategies are appropriate to ensure that the measure contains the desired content. However, in the final analysis the assessment of face and content validity is, with rare exceptions, based on the opinion of experts. Since "old boy" networks are the norm in most academic disciplines, in that we associate with people who think like we do (i.e., correctly), these must be regarded as weak tests of validity.

CRITERION VALIDITY

As we indicated, measures of validity based on expert judgments are regarded in general as weak tests of validity. Perhaps the strongest approach to validity is the assessment of **criterion validity**, which involves comparison with a "gold standard." In turn, this is divided into two forms that differ only in time. If the comparison is made at the same time (i.e., both measures are administered together) the approach is called **concurrent validity**. If the measure is used to predict future status, such as confirmation of a disease at autopsy or admission to hospital, it is called **predictive validity**. The index of criterion validity is most often a correlation coefficient between the scores on the new test and on the old (or predicted) one.

The comparison of blood pressure reading with a mercury sphygmomanometer with arterial blood pressures is an example that highlights both the use of a "gold standard" and the reason for developing a new measure, namely, reduced cost or risk. However, such true "gold standards" are difficult to come by, and one is frequently left in the situation of comparing the new measure with another better accepted, but arguably inferior measure of the same attribute. One example of this is the measurement of depression. Although new measures proliferate, nearly all are compared with one of two scales — the Beck Depression Inventory or the CES-D scale. Since both standards are short and cheap, the only reason to develop a new measure is that it will be better; however, this is difficult to prove by simply comparing with existing measures. Under these circumstances the expected correlation of the two measures should be high, but one would not anticipate correlations too close to unity; if it were nearly 1.0, the two tests are measuring almost exactly the same thing and there is little reason to develop the new one.

CONSTRUCT VALIDITY

Probably the most frequently applied, but poorest understood measure of validity is called **construct validity**. It is used in circumstances in which there is no other measure of the attribute under study. Instead of testing the relationship between the new measure and some other measure of the same thing, we invoke a theoretical construct that describes the relationship between the attribute under scrutiny and other attributes. We then examine the relation between these two measures, and if it is in the expected direction, we have evidence that both the measure and the hypothetical construct were right. However, if there is no relationship between the two measures, we have no way of determining whether our measure or our theory was wrong.

For example, if we are developing a measure of quality of life of patients with rheumatoid arthritis, we might hypothesize that the measure is strongly related to measures of function like morning stiffness or walk time, and relatively poorly related to measures of disease process like joint counts or sedimentation rate. Further, since we would hope that it is a relatively pure measure of the effect of the particular disease on perceived quality of life, we may further hypothesize that scores are uncorrelated with measures of depression. Finally, we can examine hypotheses about differences between groups, for example, that inpatients are likely to score poorer than outpatients.

It is evident that in the construct validity game there is no single study or hypothesis that clinches the case. Some hypotheses will be right and some will be wrong. Rather, the judgment of validity depends on the *weight* of the evidence being in the expected direction.

MEASUREMENT BIAS

In the previous section on research methodology we described how incorrect conclusions may result from design flaws. Biases such as the Berkson's or Neymann bias can yield estimates that are systematically higher or lower than the true value.

Unfortunately, research design errors are not the only source of bias. Large distortions can result from biases in measurement. There are innumerable sources of measurement bias; many psychologists have made careers out of cataloging how people can be induced to distort their estimates one way or another. One of the most disturbing examples derives from choices resembling the following:

> "You are responsible for the care of 100 patients who have a fatal disease. You are given a choice between two drugs: Drug A has a 60 percent chance of saving everyone; Drug B will save 60 of the 100 patients. Which will you choose?"

Under these circumstances, most subjects choose Drug B. However, the question can be framed in the logically equivalent way:

> "You are responsible for the care of 100 patients with a fatal disease. You are given a choice between two drugs. Drug A has a 40 percent chance of killing all of the patients. Drug B will result in the death of 40 of the 100 patients. Which will you choose?"

When the question is framed in this way, most respondents choose Drug A. Obviously the way a question is asked can lead to radically different responses. There are many other ways that data can be willingly or unwillingly distorted by unsuspecting investigators. Our purpose will be served by illustrating a few.

However, before we illustrate a few different kinds of bias, let's distinguish between two concepts — bias and random error. **Bias** is a *systematic* deviation from the correct value of a particular variable. The effect of bias is to distort the estimate of that variable, for example, to increase the sample mean or decrease the prevalence of some trait. In **random error**, on the other hand, there is also a deviation from the true value, but because it is random the deviation sometimes adds to the estimate and sometimes takes from it. In the long run (i.e., with a lot of subjects) these deviations cancel each other out. The effect is to increase the variability of the scores, but random error does not affect the estimate of the variable. For this reason random error can be dealt with by statistics. Since bias is a *consistent* distortion from the true value, it cannot be corrected by any statistical manipulation, and thus is more insidious.

DIAGNOSTIC SUSPICION BIAS

Under certain circumstances the rate of occurrence of a diagnosis can depart from expectations simply because of an enhanced index of suspicion on the part of the diagnostician. This bias may be highly individualized and short term. One well-documented bias of individuals is illustrated by the clinical anecdote that goes something like this: "The funniest thing happened. Saturday night in the ER I diagnosed the first case of Somaliland Camelbite Fever I've seen in 20 years. This week I saw four more cases in my office. There must be a real epidemic going around!" A more likely explanation is the *availability bias*. The one case in the ER is readily available in memory, and is likely to be recalled when anything similar comes along.

A more long-term and widespread diagnostic suspicion bias is the *syn-drome syndrome*. Over the decades it is easy to show how the popularity of certain diseases has waxed and waned. In the 1920s a common syndrome was "self-pollution", or masturbation. The clinical syndrome was well des-cribed, and there were literally institutions filled with depraved little self-polluters. In fact, W.K. Kellogg ran a sanatorium for these lost souls in Battle Creek.

Lest you feel this is a perversion of the early days of medicine prior to the advent of sophisticated diagnostic procedures, there are many current examples. Alzheimer's disease has apparently reached epidemic propor-tions. Some of the increased incidence is a result of better diagnostic tools and more old people around to get it. Nevertheless the syndrome was first described in the early 1900s. Presumably, until recently doddery old ladies were simply passed off as doddery old ladies. Now, if anyone over 65 forgets where they left their car keys, Alzheimer's is the first diagnosis to spring to mind.

We also alluded to the ureaformaldehyde foam insulation (UFFI) issue earlier. The interesting tale about UFFI is that it was installed for several decades in Europe prior to its arrival in North America. Once here, relatively few problems arose until the media announced all the lethal consequences of the stuff. Following that point physicians everywhere were diagnosing any number of complaints, from headaches to ingrown toenails, as result-ing from UFFI poisoning.

In the *Preface* we mentioned one study in which physicians "found" tonsillitis requiring surgery in about 45 percent of kids, even when two other sets of physicians declared the kids clean (or at least not ill). Here again, the expectation of finding a disorder biased what was seen.

SOCIAL DESIRABILITY BIAS

Personality psychologists now routinely include a **social desirability** scale in many of their measures. The notion is that people, when asked sensitive questions about, for example, alcohol consumption or sexual practices, will consciously or unconsciously bias their responses toward the socially acceptable answer. If the bias is deliberate and conscious, it is called "faking good," and if unconscious, "social desirability." In either case the results are the same — an underestimate of the true prevalence of undesir-able behaviors.

Several techniques have been developed to detect the presence of social desirability and to fix it if present. Many psychological scales contain imbedded social desirability scales; for example, only saints can truthfully answer "true" to the statement "I have never stolen anything." Alternatively methods such as the random response technique are designed to elicit better measures of the prevalance of unacceptable behaviors.

C.R.A.P. DETECTORS

C.R.A.P. DETECTOR III-1

Question   An investigation of the usefulness of exercise ECGs was con-ducted using patients who had been admitted to a coronary care unit (CCU). The ECG was compared with findings from coronary angiography — a very expensive and risky procedure. For obvious reasons the researchers had difficulty recruiting a large number of "normal" subjects to undergo angiography. So they took 80 men off the street, did ECGs on them (which were normal of course), assumed that they would have normal angiograms, and added them to the negative ECG-negative angiogram category. The results looked very good indeed: sensitivity was 64 percent and specificity was 93 percent. Subsequent applications of exercise ECGs in ambulatory settings have shown that it is not what it was cracked up to be, and show a sensitivity of only 33 percent. Why does the discrepancy exist?

Answer   The authors did two things to ensure that the results would look favorable. First, the positive cases were chosen from a highly select group of men in a CCU with confirmed cardiac disease, so they were more extreme than the usual suspected arteriosclerosis. Second, the initial study had too high a prevalence of disease. By including the "normal" volunteers and, better still, assuming that they had normal angiograms, they succeeded in messing the base rates in their favor.

Beware the "sample samba." By dancing around with prevalence, or by selecting extreme groups (e.g., phys. ed. students and 70-year-olds on their third myocardial infarction), anyone can make any test in the world look good.

C.R.A.P. DETECTOR III-2

Question   A recent reanalysis was conducted of the Blair et al. National Cancer Institute study of the occupational effects of formaldehyde on cancer. They were unable to show any significant relationship between formaldehyde level and lung cancer, but did demonstrate a relationship between job class and cancer. They concluded that the retrospective measurement of formaldehyde was too crude, and that blue collar workers suffered more lung cancer as a result of occupational exposure to formaldehyde. The study was not published (thank goodness!). Why?

Answer   The measurement of formaldehyde level may have been crude, but the use of job class as a surrogate for exposure ignores the many other variables that go along with job class. First, blue collar workers smoke more, and smoking causes lung cancer. Second, lower social class folks suffer more disease of all types, and live less long than upper class folks.

Correlation is not equal to causation. (See *Assessing Causation*).

C.R.A.P. DETECTOR III-3

Question In a study of the causes of cervical cancer one potential cause under investigation was whether or not the man was circumcised. The researchers approached 166 males and asked whether they were circumcised. This was then confirmed by a physical examination. Of the 44 men who said they were, 21 (48 percent) were not, and of the 122 men who said they were not circumcised, 50 (40 percent) were! Don't men know whether or not they are circumcised?

Answer Self-report may be a lousy lab test. If an investigator is using self-report data, there should be some assurance (other than faith!) that the data are valid.

C.R.A.P. DETECTOR III-4

Question For about two decades, patient management problems (PMPs) have been used as a component in the certification examination used to license physicians in Canada and the U.S. These are written simulations of a patient, on which the candidate selects options on history, physical, laboratory, and management and is rewarded (or punished) on the basis of the good options he selected and harmful options he avoided. Many studies demonstrated that candidates felt the method to be life-like (face validity), and care was taken to ensure that they were medically accurate (content validity). They have also been used as a measure of problem-solving skills. This was confirmed by a low correlation of PMP results with tests of knowledge, which suggested that they were measuring "something else" (construct validity). Can PMPs be considered to be good predictors of physician performance?

Answer Recent studies showed a very low reliability of the scores, which suggests that the "something else" they were measuring was simply noise. Other studies showed that candidates do about twice as much of everything (such as ordering lab tests) on the written problem as they do in real life. Both licensing bodies have subsequently dropped the requirement for performance on PMPs.

Face and content validity are poor substitutes for empiric forms of validity. Anyone can recruit some friends who will like his/her measure. The best test of validity is criterion-related validity. All others are relatively weak approximations.

REFERENCES

ISSUES IN CHOOSING A MEASURE

Lord Kelvin. Quoted in: Sears FW, Zemansky MW. College physics: mechanics, heat and sound. Reading, MA: Addison-Wesley, 1952.

MEASUREMENT WITH CATEGORICAL VARIABLES

Doll R, Peto R. The causes of cancer. Oxford: Oxford University Press, 1981.

Lipid Research Clinics Program. The Lipid Research Clinics coronary prevention trial results. JAMA 1984; 251:351-374.

Wynder EL, Graham EA. Tobacco smoking as a possible etiologic factor in bronchogenic carcinoma: a study of 684 proved cases. JAMA 1950; 143:329-336.

Diagnostic Tests

Cohen J. Weighted kappa: nominal scale agreement with provision for scaled disagreement or partial credit. Psychol Bull 1968; 70:213-220.

Lusted L. Medical decision making. Springfield: CC Thomas, 1968.

Meehl PE, Rosen A. Antecedent probability and the efficiency of psychometric signs, patterns, or cutting scores. Psychol Bull 1955; 52:194-216.

Polesky HF. Serologic testing to human immunodeficiency virus. MMWR 1986; 36:833.

MEASUREMENT WITH CONTINUOUS VARIABLES

American Psychological Association. Standards for educational and psychological testing. 3rd ed. Washington: APA, 1985.

Crowne DP, Marlowe D. A new scale of social desirability independent of psychopathology. J Consult Psychol 1960; 24:349-354.

Eraker SA, Sox HC. Assessment of patients' preferences for therapeutic outcomes. Med Decis Making 1981; 1:29-39.

Warner SL. Randomized response: a survey technique for eliminating evasive answer bias. J Am Stat Assoc 1965; 60:63-69.

C.R.A.P. DETECTORS

Blair A. Mortality among workers exposed to formaldehyde. J Natl Cancer Inst 1985; 75:1039-1047.

Goldschlager N, Selzer A, Cohn K. Treadmill stress tests as indicators of presence and severity of coronary artery disease. Ann Intern Med 1976; 85:277-286.

Dunn JE, Buell P. Association of cervical cancer with circumcision of sexual partner. J Natl Cancer Inst 1959; 22:749-764.

McGuire CH, Babbott D. Simulation technique in the measurement of problem-solving skills. J Educ Meas 1967; 4:1-10.

TO READ FURTHER

MEASUREMENT WITH CATEGORICAL VARIABLES

McMahon B, Pugh TF. Epidemiology: principles and methods. Boston: Little, Brown, 1970.

Diagnostic Tests

McNeil BJ, Hanley JA. Statistical approaches to the analysis of receiver operating characteristic (ROC) curves. Med Decis Making 1984; 4:137-150.
Sackett DL, Haynes RB, Tugwell P. Clinical epidemiology: a basic science for clinical medicine. Boston: Little, Brown, 1985.

MEASUREMENT WITH CONTINUOUS VARIABLES

Anastasi A. Psychological testing. 5th ed. New York: Macmillan, 1982.
Kahnemann D, Slovic P, Tversky A. Judgment under uncertainty: heuristics and biases. Cambridge: Cambridge University Press, 1982.
Norman GR, Streiner DL. PDQ statistics. Toronto: BC Decker, 1986.
Norman GR, Streiner DL. Principles of measurement in health sciences. Oxford: Oxford University Press, 1989.

ASSESSING CAUSATION

In this final chapter we will look at how epidemiologists attempt to establish causation, that is, to decide whether factor A can possibly be the cause of disorder or state B. Perhaps the earliest rules for assessing causation were Koch's Postulates, which were set forth about a century ago for determining whether an infectious agent is the cause of a disease:

1. Every diseased person (or animal) must have the organism;
2. It must be possible to isolate the organism and grow it in a pure culture;
3. A susceptible host, when inoculated with the organism, must develop the disease; and
4. The organism must be recoverable from the newly infected host.

While these could easily be applied to acute infectious diseases, there are many situations in which the rules do not apply. Sir Bradford Hill proposed a variation of these criteria that covers a greater variety of situations, which has been used with little modification ever since. These nine criteria, listed in descending order of importance, are:

1. The **strength** of the association;
2. The **consistency** of the association;
3. Its **specificity**;
4. The **temporal** relationship;
5. The **biologic** gradient;
6. Biologic **plausibility**;
7. **Coherence**;
8. Evidence from **experimentation**; and
9. **Analogy**.

We will use these criteria to examine one theory of the etiology of multiple sclerosis (MS). Multiple sclerosis is in many ways an intriguing disease. One of the most puzzling aspects is its geographic distribution; the prevalence seems to be directly proportional to distance from the equator. The disorder is far more common in the northern parts of North America and the southern parts of Australia and New Zealand than it is in the tropics. However, just to make things a bit more interesting, MS is quite rare in Japan, a country at the same latitude as California.

A number of etiologic theories have been proposed that try to account for this distribution of MS. These have ranged from a genetic predisposition to the disorder, to dietary factors, to exposure, and to canine excrement. One group of theories holds that MS is caused by a viral agent, possibly even a slow virus (a class of viruses frequently invoked by researchers whenever the relationship between exposure and outcome is not readily apparent). In this chapter we will focus on one viral theory, exposure to the measles virus, to see whether it is a plausible explanation.

THE CRITERIA

STRENGTH OF ASSOCIATION

This criterion holds that the stronger the association between the supposed cause and the effect, the greater the chances are that a causal relationship exists. In this example there should be a higher rate of multiple sclerosis among people who have been exposed to the measles virus than among those who have not been exposed. Conversely, measles antibody titers may be higher in MS patients than in people who do not have the disease.

The data in this regard are tantalizing, but unfortunately they are also inconclusive (this can cynically be called the "So what else is new?" effect in epidemiology). Adams and Imagawa found that various measles antibody titers were higher in MS patients than in normals. However, as can be seen in Table 4-1, the magnitude of the difference is not overly large in this study or in later ones, although a trend is definitely present. Thus, on the basis of this criterion, the case for causality is not ruled out, but does seem somewhat weak.

CONSISTENCY OF ASSOCIATION

The association between the suspected cause and the outcome should be seen across numerous studies, ideally by different research teams, in different settings, and under different circumstances. The larger the number of studies that demonstrate such a relationship, the stronger the evidence. There have been about 35 such studies conducted since 1962, and higher titers of measles antibodies were found in MS patients in all but four of them. So this criterion would lend support to a causal hypothesis involving exposure to measles.

TABLE 4–1   Percent of Subjects Over or Under 32 on the Serum Dilution Test for Measles Virus

Reciprocal of Serum Dilution		MS Patients	Controls
	< 32	64	86
	> 32	36	14

However, in and of itself consistency does not *prove* association, much less causation. (Indeed, none of the criteria proves causation; they can only be used either to strengthen or to weaken the case for it.) All of the studies can suffer from the same types of bias, or the association can be in the opposite direction. For example, a number of studies showed that the use of conjugated estrogens was associated with a much higher risk of endometrial carcinoma. However, Horwitz and Feinstein pointed out that all of the studies suffered from the same type of sampling bias: women were identified on the basis of vaginal bleeding. Estrogens may cause bleeding, which leads to an intensive work-up during which the cancer is discovered. It is possible (indeed, they found it probable) that endometrial cancer is almost as prevalent in the general population, but women who did not take estrogens didn't have the symptom of vaginal bleeding, and so their cancer was not detected (see the discussion on subject selection biases in *Threats to Validity*). When the bias was eliminated, the odds ratio dropped from 11.98 to 1.7, or in essence from a twelvefold risk of developing cancer for women who have used estrogens to less than a twofold risk.

SPECIFICITY OF ASSOCIATION

Ideally, the cause should lead to only one outcome, and that outcome should result from that single cause (Fig. 4-1). Unfortunately, life is rarely this simple. Obviously not everyone who gets measles later develops MS; measles can lead to a host of other adverse outcomes (including sterility), and it is quite possible that MS is multidetermined and has other causes (e.g., genetic predisposition, exposure to other viruses). To use another example, obesity increases the risk not only for stroke, but also for diabetes; however, both diabetes and stroke can arise from causes other than obesity.

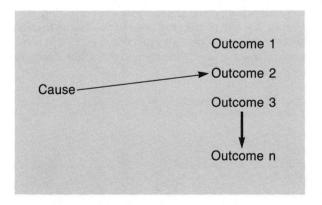

Figure 4-1 Ideal specificity of association.

When specificity does exist it can be a very powerful argument for causality. For example, the annual rate of malignant mesothelioma is extremely low, averaging fewer than three cases per million for males and about 1.4 cases per million for females. The incidence of mesothelioma among asbestos workers, however, is 100 to 200 times higher. It has also been estimated that there was exposure to asbestos in at least 85 percent of the mesothelioma cases; indeed, even this very high figure may be an underestimate, since families of asbestos workers are at risk through fibers brought home on clothing. It would seem from this evidence that there is a high degree of specificity, because exposure to asbestos is found in nearly all cases of mesothelioma.

Thus, if there is specificity of association, it strengthens the case for causality. However, a lack of specificity does not necessarily weaken the case.

TEMPORALITY OF ASSOCIATION

For factor A to cause outcome B, A must precede B (Fig. 4-2). That is, the person must have been exposed to the putative cause before the onset of the disorder. While this may appear so self-evident that it hardly bears mentioning, it is indeed difficult to establish in many cases, especially for chronic conditions with long latency periods. In the case of MS and measles it is obvious that the *clinical onset* of measles precedes that of MS; however, it would have to be shown that MS did not have a long, insidious onset that may have begun *before* the person contracted measles.

To use a different example, a number of studies demonstrated that a low serum cholesterol level was associated with a higher risk of cancer, which led some to postulate that a low cholesterol level somehow results in cancer. Recently, however, Dyer showed that the more likely explanation is that undetected cancer leads to a lowering of the cholesterol level. Thus, the purported "cause," cholesterol level, may actually occur *after* what was supposed to be the "effect," cancer.

One field particularly prone to problems in interpreting temporality is psychiatry, especially with respect to those studies that try to uncover family patterns that predispose people to major disorders. Since many problems manifest themselves only when the patient is in his/her 20s or 30s, the vast

Figure 4-2 Temporality of association.

majority of studies use either retrospective case-series or case-control designs. The assumption made is that any family dynamics uncovered were present prior to the onset of the disorder. For example, the supposed etiology of early infantile autism was once thought to be the emotional coldness and withdrawal of the parents, and especially of the mother. However, later studies indicated that these attributes were more likely the parents' reactions to an unresponsive infant, rather than the cause, thereby supporting what parents have long maintained: insanity is inherited — we get it from our children.

BIOLOGIC GRADIENT

The biologic gradient, or dose-response relationship, states that if more exposure leads to more of the disease, the case for causality is strengthened. This would imply that those who had more severe cases of measles should be more likely to develop MS, or to develop more serious symptoms earlier on. The evidence in this regard, however, is lacking. The biologic gradient is seen most clearly with regard to toxins and carcinogens. Newhouse, for instance, cited data gathered by Merewether and Prince that showed the relationship between length of employment in the asbestos industry and the incidence of fibrosis. The data look something like Figure 4-3. There seems to be a definite trend, in that longer exposure to asbestos results in a greater proportion of people who develop fibrosis.

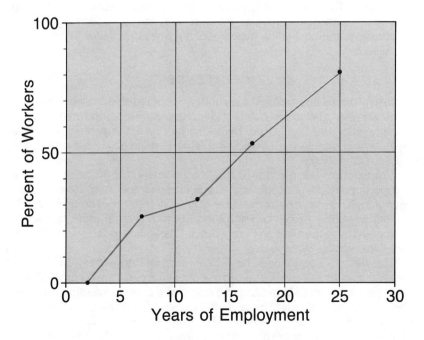

Figure 4-3 Length of employment in asbestos industry versus incidence of fibrosis.

For less obvious causal relationships there may be an amount of a toxic agent below which there are no adverse effects (at least none that we can measure with our current technology), and a ceiling, whereby no further increase leads to a greater effect. Some people postulate this is the case with ionizing radiation; there is no increased risk for cancer if exposure is below a certain threshold, whereas death is a certainty above an upper limit. Between these upper and lower limits, however, there may be a dose-response relationship.

BIOLOGIC PLAUSIBILITY

If the association makes sense from the perspective of biology, there is a (somewhat) greater plausibility, if not probability, of a causal relationship. Thus, although the etiology of MS is still unknown, there is evidence from related disorders that viral infections, and especially measles, can result in demyelination in the central nervous system. For example, high measles antibody titers are found in the serum and cerebrospinal fluid of patients with subacute sclerosing panencephalitis. This would indicate that a causal relationship between measles and MS is at least within the bounds of possibility.

However, a lack of plausibility may simply reflect our incomplete knowledge of physiology and biology. Until recently no known mechanism existed to explain how psychological stress could result in a greater susceptibility to infectious diseases and cancer. Only within the past few years has it been shown that stress may produce immune suppression by affecting immune cell function. As was the case with the criterion of specificity, plausibility strengthens the hypothesis, but a lack of plausibility does not weaken it.

COHERENCE

When discussing biologic plausibility, we noted that the absence of a plausible explanation was not necessarily damning to a good theory; it may simply reflect our ignorance. By the same token, the postulated causal relationship should not conflict with what *is* generally known about the disease or disorder.

For example, we mentioned that the prevalence of MS seemed to be proportional to the latitude, with some exceptions in Asia. However, the geographic distribution of measles is, if anything, opposite to what one would want; it is more common in the tropics than in more temperate climates. Using the criterion of coherence, this would argue against a causal link between the two diseases.

Needless to say, theories have been proposed to explain this inverse relationship. It has been postulated that subacute cases are common below tha age of 15 years in the tropics, and that this early infection provides protection against later, more serious ones. This may be taken as an example of Edington's Theory: "The number of different hypotheses erected to explain a given biologic phenomenon is inversely proportional to the available knowledge."

EXPERIMENTAL EVIDENCE

In some cases there may be experimental evidence that can show a causal relationship. This evidence can be of many types: "true" experiments in the lab, randomized trials, animal models, experiments in nature, or interventions in which some preventative action is taken.

An experiment in nature would exist if a place were found where MS had been nonexistent until the society was introduced to the many benefits of civilization, including measles. This may indeed have been the case in the Faroe Islands. MS suddenly appeared in 1943, with 24 of 25 of the known cases first appearing between then and 1960, which is consistent with a mean age of onset of about 25 years. This "epidemic" coincided with the invasion of Denmark by Germany in 1940, and the subsequent stationing of about 800 British troops on the islands 4 days later. Although not conclusive evidence in its own right, this naturalistic experiment strengthens the case for MS being caused by some form of infectious agent.

Since an effective vaccine for measles was introduced to North America in 1963, there has been a dramatic decline in the prevalence of subacute sclerosing panencephalitis. If there is a causal relationship between measles and MS, we should begin to see a similar drop in MS starting about 25 to 30 years later, or some time around 1990. This would be an example of experimental evidence from an intervention. In this case, as in many others, the treatment was not predicated on an assumed relationship between the cause and effect; the aim of vaccination was simply to eliminate measles, not MS. Any evidence of a reduction in the incidence of MS would be a side benefit, probably unanticipated at the time the vaccination program began.

Experimental evidence again strengthens (but does not necessarily prove) causation. However, as with most of these criteria, its absence does not weaken the case because it is often extremely difficult or unethical to do the types of studies that would yield less equivocal results.

ANALOGY

The weakest form of evidence regarding causality is arguing from an analogy. Returning again to the example of measles and subacute sclerosing panencephalitis, we can state that just as measles can cause one form of demyelinating disorder, it is reasonable to expect that it can cause another.

In this regard analogy is very similar to biologic plausibility. For this reason, some authors don't distinguish between the two and drop this last category from the list of criteria for causality.

SUMMARY

Even if a theory passes all these criteria with flying colors, it does not necessarily *prove* causation beyond any shadow of a doubt. However, the more criteria that are met (especially the ones near the top of the list), the more likely it is that the causal hypothesis is in the right ball park, given the current state of our knowledge. Newer discoveries, however, may cause us to modify or even discard our cause-effect theory, and to replace it with a different one. Buck notes that we would prefer a new hypothesis to a well-established one only if it meets at least one of the following criteria:

1. The new hypothesis makes more precise predictions than the old one;
2. More observations are explainable with the new hypothesis;
3. Previous observations are explained in more detail;
4. The new hypothesis has passed tests that the older hypothesis has failed;
5. It suggests tests or makes predictions not made by the older hypothesis; or
6. It has unified or connected phenomena not previously considered to be related.

Thus any causal hypothesis should be seen as just that, a hypothesis that accounts for what we know now, but that may be modified or overturned at any time.

C.R.A.P. DETECTORS

C.R.A.P. DETECTOR IV-1

Question Ney used the statistic that the "rate of increase in child abuse parallels the rate of increase in abortions" to argue against abortions. Although he didn't calculate it, the correlation between the number of abortions and the number of cases of alleged physical ill treatment in Ontario between 1971 and 1977 is 0.85. Does this high correlation support Ney's case for a causal association?

Answer One of the cardinal rules of statistics is that you can't draw causation from a correlation. In fact, we calculated that the correlation between the number of child abuse cases and the number of high school graduates during the same period is 0.86, and between cases of abuse and the gross revenue of Canadian railroads is 0.92. Nobody would argue, however, that the way to curb child abuse is to cut enrolment in high schools, or to make the railroads lose money.

A nice demonstration that strong correlation does not necessarily imply any meaningful relationship is shown in Figure 4-4, which plots the number of wins in 1984 by teams in the American Football Conference as a function of the number of letters in the team name. The correlation between these two variables is 0.70, a figure high enough to cause most researchers to have dreams of tenure.

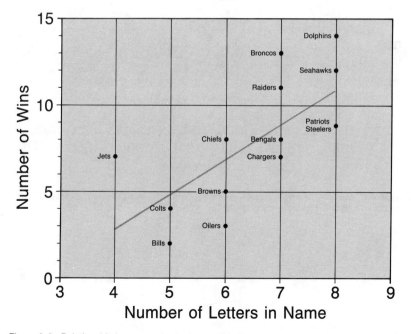

Figure 4-4 Relationship between wins by football teams and number of letters in their names.

C.R.A.P. DETECTOR IV-2

Question   There has been concern expressed recently that the low rate of infection from measles has caused parents to become complacent and not have their children immunized. The fear is that there will be an outbreak of measles, with the attending death rate that used to characterize the infection. Is this a concern? Was the vaccine responsible for the marked reduction in the case fatality rate from measles?

Answer   Not according to McKeown. Figure 4-5, based on the graph in his book, *The Modern Rise of Population*, shows that the decline in the mortality rate from measles among children began long before the immunization program was initiated. This reflects the importance of establishing a temporal relationship before anything can be said about a causal one.

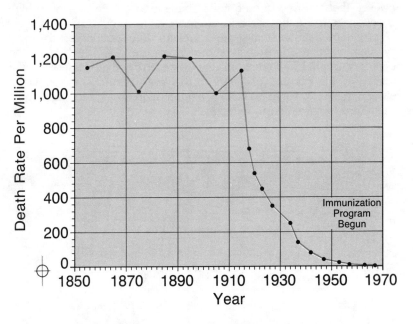

Figure 4-5 Mortality rate from measles over time. Data from McKeown T. The modern rise of population. London: Edward Arnold, 1976:96.

C.R.A.P. DETECTOR IV-3

Question   A group of researchers in England found that bus drivers had a higher rate of coronary heart disease than did conductors. One hypothesis put forward to explain this was that conductors had to run up and down the stairs of the double-decker buses, whereas the drivers spent all day on their (and the buses') seats. Thus, it may be that a more sedentary job increases the risk of heart disease. Is this a viable explanation for their results?

Answer   Only if all other differences between drivers and conductors are ruled out. The same research group compared the body builds of the two groups by doing an "epidemiologic survey" of their uniforms! As Figure 4-6 shows, a larger proportion of drivers than conductors had trouser waists of 36 inches or more, irrespective of age. So it would appear that there may have been constitutional differences between the groups from the very beginning, which makes an interpretation based on other group differences chancy at best.

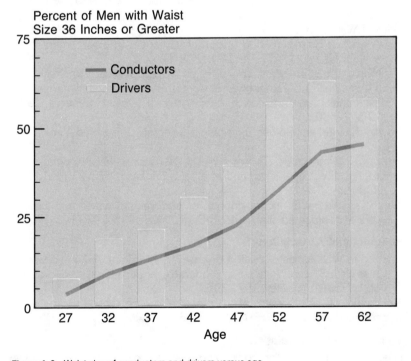

Figure 4-6   Waist size of conductors and drivers versus age.

REFERENCES

Fletcher RH, Fletcher SW, Wagner EH. Clinical epidemiology: the essentials. Baltimore: Williams & Wilkins, 1982.

Hill AB. The environment and disease: association or causation? Proc R Soc Med 1965; 58:295-300.

Whitaker JN. What causes the disease? In: Scheinberg LC, ed. Multiple sclerosis. New York: Raven Press, 1983:7.

THE CRITERIA

Strength of Association

Adams JM, Imagawa D. Measles antibodies in multiple sclerosis. Proc Soc Exp Biol Med 1962; 111:562-566.

Consistency of Association

Gray LA, Christopherson WM, Hoover RN. Estrogens and endometrial carcinoma. Obstet Gynecol 1977; 49:385-389.

Horwitz RI, Feinstein AR. Alternative analytic methods for case-control studies of estrogens and endometrial cancer. N Engl J Med 1978; 299:1089-1094.

Mack TM, Pike MC, Henderson BE, Pfeffer RI, Gerkins VR, Arthur M, Brown SE. Estrogens and endometrial cancer in a retirement community. N Engl J Med 1976; 294:1262-1267.

McDonald TW, Annegers JF, O'Fallon WM, Dockerty MB, Malkasian GD, Kurland LT. Exogenous estrogen and endometrial carcinoma: case-control and incidence study. Am J Obstet Gynecol 1977; 127:572-580.

Norrby E. Viral antibodies in multiple sclerosis. Prog Med Virol 1978; 24:1-39.

Smith DC, Prentice R, Thompson DJ, Herrmann WL. Association of exogenous estrogens and endometrial carcinoma. N Engl J Med 1975; 293:1164-1167.

Ziel HK, Finkle WD. Increased risk of endometrial carcinoma among users of conjugated estrogens. N Engl J Med 1975; 293:1167-1170.

Specificity of Association

Buchanan WD. Asbestos-related diseases: I. Introduction. In: Michaels L, Chissick SS, eds. Asbestos: properties, applications, and hazards. Vol. 1. New York: Wiley, 1979:395.

McDonald JC, McDonald AD. Epidemiology of mesothelioma from estimated incidence. Prev Med 1977; 6:426-446.

Temporality of Association

Dyer AR. A method for combining results from several prospective epidemiological studies. Stat Med 1986; 5:303-317.

Eisenberg L. The fathers of autistic children. Am J Orthopsychiatry 1957; 27:715-724.

Eisenberg L, Kanner L. Early infantile autism 1943-55. Am J Orthopsy-
    chiatry 1956; 26:556-566.
Pitfield M, Oppenheim AN. Child rearing attitudes of mothers of psychotic
    children. J Child Psychol Psychiatry 1964; 5:51-57.

Biologic Gradient

Newhouse M. Asbestos-related diseases: IV. Epidemiology of asbestos-
    related disease. In: Michaels L, Chissick SS, eds. Asbestos: properties,
    applications, and hazards. Vol. 1. New York: Wiley, 1979: 465.

Biologic Plausibility

Marx JL. The immune system "belongs in the body." Science 1985;
    227:1190-1192.
ter Meulen V, Stephenson JR. The possible role of viral infections in
    multiple sclerosis and other related demyelinating diseases. In: Hallpike
    JF, Adams CWM, Tourtellotte WW, eds. Multiple sclerosis: pathol- '
    ogy, diagnosis and management. London: Chapman & Hall, 1983:241.

Coherence

Bloch A. Murphy's law, and other reasons why things go wrong. Los
    Angeles: Price/Stern/Sloan, 1979.
Carp RI, Warner HB, Merz GS. Viral etiology of multiple sclerosis. Prog
    Med Virol 1978; 24:158-177.

Experimental Evidence

Bloch AB, Orenstein WA, Wassilak SG, Stetler HC, Turner PM, Amler
    RW, Bart KJ, Hinman AR. Epidemiology of measles and its complica-
    tions. In: Gruenberg EM, Lewis C, Goldston SE, eds. Vaccinating
    against brain syndromes: the campaign against measles and rubella.
    New York: Oxford University Press, 1986:5.
Kurtzke JF, Hyllested K. Multiple sclerosis in the Faroe Islands: I. Clinical
    and epidemiological features. Ann Neurol 1979; 5:6-21.

Summary

Buck C. Popper's philosophy for epidemiologists. Internat J Epidemiol
    1975; 4:159-168.

C.R.A.P. DETECTORS

McKeown T. The modern rise of population. London: Edward Arnold,
    1976.
Morris JN, Heady JA, Raffle PAB. Physique of London busmen:
    epidemiology of uniforms. Lancet, Sept. 15, 1956; 569-570.
Morris JN, Heady JA, Raffle PAB, Roberts CG, Parks JW. Coronary
    heart-disease and physical activity of work. Lancet, Nov. 21, 1953;
    1053-1057.
Ney P. Relationship between abortion and child abuse. Can J Psychiatry
    1979; 24:10-20.

TO READ FURTHER

Department of Clinical Epidemiology and Biostatistics. How to read clinical journals: IV. To determine etiology or causation. Can Med Assoc J 1981; 124:985-990.

Hill AB. The environment and disease: association or causation? Proc R Soc Med 1965; 58:295-300.

APPENDIX

A Brief Epidemish-English Dictionary

In the course of writing their reports and journal articles, researchers in epidemiology often use words or phrases whose meanings are somewhat obscure. To assist the reader in understanding these terms (and to provide a little amusement), we provide herewith a brief dictionary.

To begin, we offer the definition of clinical epidemiology (itself an obscure term), which is credited to Dr. Stephen Leader of the University of Sydney:

"Clinical epidemiology is that branch of alchemy whose goal it is to turn bulls--t into airline tickets."

And now to the dictionary:

When The Researcher Says	*He/She Really Means*
A trend was noted.	The statistical test was not significant.
The demographic characteristics of the nonresponders were similar to those of the rest of the sample.	All we really had on them was age and sex.
Agreement between the raters was acceptable.	The agreement was so bad that we don't dare to include the actual number in the paper.
The questionnaire was circulated to a panel of experts to establish face validity.	Our friends liked it...and the bottle of scotch we included.
The rate of lung cancer among the hourly rate employees was significantly higher, which may be caused by excess PBCP exposure.	It might also be caused by obvious things like smoking and social class, but I'm interested in PBCPs today.
In a case series of 12 patients nine showed clinically significant improvement on the experimental drug.	With the help of the drug company representative, I judged which patients got better under my care.
The correlation was highly significant ($p < 0.0001$).	With 10,000 subjects, *any* correlation is highly significant.

The response rate was 60 percent, which is acceptable for studies of this type.

However, the study itself was so bad that even a 100 percent response rate wouldn't have saved it.

Although there was no overall difference in mortality, the rate of left clavicular cancer was higher in blue-eyed females in the exposed group.

If you look at enough things, sooner or later one of them is bound to turn out to be significantly different.

While the results appear to be consistent with the predictions, further research is warranted.

I've already applied for a new grant this year.

Further research is required to clarify the results.

I haven't a clue what it all means.

The difference was statistically significant ($p < 0.0001$).

...but clinically useless.

The study was a single-blind trial.

Everybody knew who was getting what except for the poor patient.

A retrospective study was conducted.

We had all these data sitting around, and needed some fast publications.

Morbidity and mortality from Blum-Streinorman's disease represents a significant burden on society.

It's my own narrow interest, but I have to justify the research somehow.

The overall agreement was 87 percent, which represents a truly remarkable rate of agreement (Kappa = 0.12).

Chance corrected agreement was so abysmal that we thought we had better talk about raw agreement.

Based on current trends, the incidence of self-pollution in the year 2000 will be...

Draw a straight line through the data from one hospital in 1970 and 1980 and that's what we got.

It is widely known that...

I can't be bothered to look up the reference.

A one-tailed test was used.

The results wouldn't be significant with a two-tailed test.

After adjusting for baseline differences between the groups...	We did a lousy job of randomizing.
After adjusting for confounders...	Boy, did these groups differ!
One possible explanation for these results is...	I can only think of one.
Forty patients agreed to participate.	The others were able to pay their hospital bills.
After conducting a pilot study, we decided to use a mailed questionnaire.	We got tired of people slamming the phone in our ear.
After conducting a pilot study, we decided to use face-to-face interviews.	They wouldn't return the mailed questionnaires either.
The data were normalized by truncating outliers.	We couldn't get the results we wanted, so we threw out subjects until we got what we were looking for.
We did not include premorbid status and number of previous hospitalizations in the model.	We forgot to gather these data.

The agreement between raters was
    excellent
    good
    acceptable
    low
	good
	fair
	nonexistent
	negative

Data was analyzed using the Schmedlap-Scheisskopf test.	We tried the usual tests but they didn't give significant results.

INDEX